Baillière's

CLINICAL ONCOLOGY

INTERNATIONAL PRACTICE AND RESEARCH

Baillière's

CLINICAL ONCOLOGY

INTERNATIONAL PRACTICE AND RESEARCH

Volume 1/Number 2
July 1987

Contemporary Palliation of Difficult Symptoms

THELMA D. BATES MB, ChB, FRCR
Guest Editor

Baillière Tindall
London Philadelphia Toronto Sydney Tokyo

Baillière Tindall 24–28 Oval Road
W.B. Saunders London NW1 7DX, UK

West Washington Square
Philadelphia, PA 19105, USA

1 Goldthorne Avenue
Toronto, Ontario M8Z 5T9, Canada

Harcourt Brace Jovanovich Group (Australia) Pty Ltd
Post Office Box 300, North Ryde, NSW 2113, Australia

Exclusive Agent in Japan:
Maruzen Co. Ltd. (Journals Division)
3–10 Nihonbashi 2-chome, Chuo-ku, Tokyo 103, Japan

ISSN 0950-3560

ISBN 0-7020-1227-0 (single copy)

Baillière's Clinical Oncology is published three times each year by Baillière Tindall. Annual subscription prices are:

TERRITORY	ANNUAL SUBSCRIPTION	SINGLE ISSUE
1. UK & Republic of Ireland	£29.50 post free	£17.50 post free
2. USA & Canada	US $55.00 post free	US $28.00 post free
3. All other countries	£37.50 post free	£19.50 post free

The editor of this publication is Seán Duggan, Baillière Tindall, 24–28 Oval Road, London NW1 7DX, UK.

Baillière's Clinical Oncology was published from 1982 to 1986 as *Clinics in Oncology*.

Typeset by Phoenix Photosetting, Chatham.
Printed and bound in Great Britain by Mackays of Chatham Ltd.

Contributors to this issue

MARY BAINES MB, BChir, Consultant Physician, St Christopher's Hospice, Lawrie Park Road, London SE26 6DZ, UK.

THELMA D. BATES MB, ChB, FRCR, Director, South East London Radiotherapy Centre; Consultant Radiotherapist and Oncologist, St Thomas' Hospital, London SE1 7EH, UK.

KENNETH C. CALMAN MD, PhD, FRCP, FRCS, FRSE, Dean of Postgraduate Medicine, University of Glasgow, Glasgow G12 8QQ, UK.

SUSAN P. CLOSS MB, MRCP, MRCPath, previously Senior Registrar, St Christopher's Hospice, Lawrie Park Road, London SE26 6DZ, UK.

MATTHEW E. CONOLLY MD, FACP, FRCP, Professor of Medicine and Pharmacology, UCLA School of Medicine, Los Angeles, CA90024, USA.

DAVID CUNNINGHAM MB, ChB, MD, MRCP, Senior Clinical Scientist, Ludwig Institute for Cancer Research, St Mary's Hospital Medical School, London W2; Honorary Consultant Medical Oncologist, St Mary's Hospital, London W2 and The Hammersmith Hospital, London W12, UK.

KENNETH C. H. FEARON MB, ChB, MD, Surgical Registrar, University Department of Surgery, Royal Infirmary, Glasgow G4 0SF, UK.

G. W. HANKS BSc, MB, MRCP, Consultant Physician and Honorary Senior Lecturer in Medicine, Royal Marsden Hospital, Fulham Road, London SW3 6JJ, UK; Institute of Cancer Research, University of London.

P. J. HOSKIN BSc, MB BS, MRCP, FRCR, Cancer Research Campaign Research Fellow and Honorary Senior Registrar, Royal Marsden Hospital, Sutton, Surrey, SM2 5PT, UK.

A. M. HOY BSc, MRCP, FRCR, Medical Director, The Princess Alice Hospice, West End Lane, Esher, Surrey, KT10 8NA; Honorary Consultant Radiotherapist and Oncologist, St Thomas' Hospital, Lambeth Palace Road, London SE1 7EH.

JENNIFER E. HUGHES BM, BCh, MRCP, MRC Psych, Senior Research Fellow, Department of Psychiatry, University of Southampton, SO9 4PE; Honorary Consultant Psychiatrist, Royal South Hants Hospital, Southampton SO9 4PE, UK.

C. F. B. REGNARD MBCLB, BMSc, Medical Director, St Oswald's Hospice, Regent Avenue, Newcastle upon Tyne NE3 1EE, UK; Honorary Associate Lecturer in Pharmacological Sciences, University of Newcastle upon Tyne.

MIKE SOUKOP MB, ChB, FRCP, Consultant Physician and Medical Oncologist, Royal Infirmary, Glasgow G4 0SF, UK.

AVERIL STEDEFORD MB, BS, DCH, DObstRCOG, DPM, MRCPsych, Consultant in Psychological Medicine, Sir Michael Sobell House, Churchill Hospital, Oxford OX3 7LJ, UK; Clinical Lecturer, Faculty of Medicine, University of Oxford.

BASIL A. STOLL FRCR, Honorary Consulting Physician, Department of Radiotherapy and Oncology, St Thomas' Hospital, London SE1 7EH, UK.

Table of contents

FORTHCOMING ISSUE

November 1987
Metastases
M. SLEVIN

RECENT ISSUE

March 1987
Bone Tumours
R. SOUHAMI

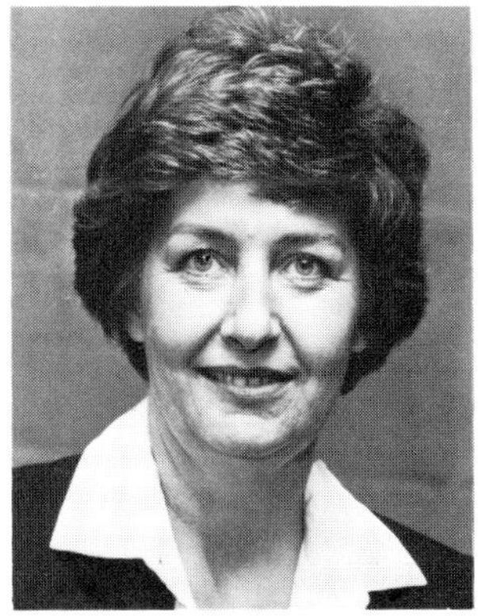

Foreword

One of the most important advances in oncology in recent years has been the rapid growth of knowledge in palliative cancer management, not least in the control of pain and other distressing symptoms. This was initiated largely by the British hospice movement and has resulted in changing attitudes to cancer palliation, as distinct from the goal of cancer cure at an earlier stage of the disease. Quality of life is now given a great deal more emphasis than it was twenty years ago.

The authors of this book—hospice physicians and oncologists—were given the brief to look in depth at a common distressing symptom or syndrome and to relate management to aetiology. A major aim was to balance advantages for the patient against disadvantages, in the framework of the modern multidisciplinary approach which includes the patient in the decision-making process.

The current generation of clinicians has had very inadequate teaching in palliative care, and subjects such as the control of severe chronic cancer pain are only just beginning to be included in undergraduate and postgraduate teaching. Fundamental to good palliation is the ability to control distressing symptoms and, as will be seen in the following chapters, contemporary palliation of symptoms has become a sophisticated art. There exists today a large body of knowledge which is still not widely taught and therefore not routinely practised. The challenge is to implement this knowledge.

THELMA D. BATES

1

The provision of good palliative care

THELMA D. BATES

Clinical effort, research and funding in cancer is, in the main, directed towards curing cancer. Of course, cancer prevention, early diagnosis and curative facilities accessible to all members of the public are essential, but there is a serious negative imbalance in the provision of palliative as opposed to curative aspects of cancer management. It is particularly important that this weakness should be redressed, for the majority of cancer patients today are not cured.

These deficiencies in palliative care exist in spite of the very considerable advances made in the last 25 years. Initiated principally by the hospice movement in the United Kingdom, these advances have not been widely used and many cancer patients still suffer unnecessarily. This book presents the most recent developments which, if implemented, would represent an important advance in cancer management.

The basic essential to good palliative care is the ability to control distressing physical symptoms. How can a patient attend fully to social, spiritual and other problems when suffering from symptoms such as unrelieved severe chronic pain or nausea? The oncologist also has to know when to start and stop active (palliative) treatment with radiotherapy, chemotherapy or surgery, and at the same time he must be able to listen and respond appropriately to his patient. The main obstacles which have to be overcome in order to improve the present low standard of palliative cancer care are:

- the negative attitude of many doctors to palliative (in contrast to curative) approaches to cancer,
- a lack of understanding of what can be achieved,
- a serious deficiency in medical education,
- a lack of research and development funding.

THE TEAM APPROACH

The goal of palliative care in patients who have cancer which cannot be cured is to improve the quality of remaining life, no matter whether its duration is a matter of weeks or many years. Palliative cancer care involves not only care and support of the patient but also an appreciation of his particular problems, together with concern and support for his family.

Palliative management pays attention to details of comfort, and often requires more time than is generally available to a busy practitioner. This lack of time can be overcome to some extent by the delegation of aspects of care to nurses and others who work closely with the doctor. Much that has been considered in the past to be the role of the doctor can be carried out by experienced nurses, especially if they are given additional training. Nurses can extend the regular review of symptoms, give guidance and support to the patient and family and provide specialist help for mastectomy, laryngectomy and stoma patients. As the end approaches, they can provide skilled terminal and bereavement care.

The team includes the physiotherapist, occupational therapist, therapy radiographer, dietitian, medical social worker and clergy. All have an important part to play in achieving maximum rehabilitation and quality of life. Those who provide a laundry and incontinence service and 'Meals on Wheels' can also be invaluable for the severely disabled. Total management involves detailed, complex care requiring a closely co-ordinated collaboration between the hospital and community personnel (Table 1) and individual circumstances will dictate whether the main co-ordinator is the oncologist or the family doctor or another.

THE SIZE OF THE PROBLEM

The size of the problem of providing adequate palliative cancer care is

Table 1. Basic palliative care personnel.

Medical	Family doctor	
	Cancer specialists	Radiotherapist
		Chemotherapist
		Surgeon
	Pain specialists	Anaesthetist
		Neurosurgeon
	Psychiatrist	
	Hospice doctor	
Nursing	Community nursing services	District nurse
		Health Visitor
		Night nurse
		Twilight nurse
	Hospital nurses	
	Specialist nurses	Oncology
		Mastectomy
		Laryngectomy
		Stomatherapy
		Hospice nurse
		Nurse counsellor
Other professionals	Physiotherapist	
	Therapy radiographer	
	Dietitian	
	Surgical appliance specialist	
	Medical social worker	
	Pharmacist	
	Chaplain	

considerable. Cancer is a common condition affecting one person in four, and responsible for one in five of all deaths. The recorded cancer incidence of 4.0 males and 3.8 females per 1000 in the population of England and Wales (Cancer Statistics Registry, 1986) is likely to be an underestimate. Despite recent advances in the curative treatment of individual tumours, the overall 'cure-rate' (however this imprecise term is measured) is no more than 20–25% (Haybittle, 1983).

In the UK, an attempt at cure is made in only about half of all cancer patients, using one or more of the three treatment modalities, surgery, radiotherapy and chemotherapy. A study of epidemiology and prognosis from the Birmingham Region Cancer Registry by Waterhouse (1974) found that in 41 236 cancer patients, only 44.7% received radical treatment which resulted in initial complete eradication of the tumour. The corrected 5-year survival rates of this group was 42.9% (males) and 55.1% (females), compared with 18.5% (males) and 34.5% (females) for all cases.

To be successful, radical treatment often has to be aggressive. It may therefore be associated with unpleasant side effects and is invariably stressful. Such treatment is clearly justified in three situations:

- when cure is possible,
- when there is a realistic chance of worthwhile prolongation of life,
- in the context of a clinical trial with the patient participating in an investigation of a new and potentially effective method of treatment.

The decision to withhold curative therapy is a crucial one and is not always easy in the individual patient. Attempts to cure the incurable are, however, not in the best interests of patients who are inevitably going to die from their cancer; these patients need palliative and not 'hopefully radical' treatment. It must be recognized that today approximately half of all cancer patients are incurable from the time of diagnosis, and of those receiving curative treatment, some 60% will show recurrence and they too will require palliative management.

Cancer includes a wide spectrum of disease patterns which are all associated with different prognoses. For example, in carcinoma of the bronchus, cure is rare, prognosis is measured in months and most patients need palliative management from the time of diagnosis. In carcinoma of the breast, although probably no more than 20% are cured, prognosis is measured in years and it is not unknown for patients to die of their disease as long as 25 years after diagnosis (Brinkley and Haybittle, 1977). Many of these patients need palliative management over a number of years, and therefore estimates of numbers of breast cancer patients requiring palliative care which are based on 5-year survival and recurrence-free rates, will underestimate the size of the problem.

In the last 25 years the hospice movement in the UK has shown that a great deal can be done to help patients who are dying from cancer and in particular they have demonstrated that severe chronic pain can usually be relieved without dulling of consciousness. A patient requiring terminal care has been defined as '. . . one in whom, following accurate diagnosis, death is certain and not too far distant and for whom treatment has changed from the curative to the palliative' (Soukop and Calman, 1977). This definition might be taken to imply that treatment aimed to cure commonly continues up to the terminal phase, when in fact, frequently it does not. Terminal care is actually the last phase of palliative care. Surely the high quality of care described in hospice literature (Saunders, 1984; Twycross and Lack, 1983 and 1986) should be a logical continuation of previous high quality palliative care and not reserved just for those who are acknowledged to be dying.

THE CONTROL OF DISTRESSING SYMPTOMS

Patients with incurable cancer may suffer from a variety of distressing symptoms caused by the disease process, its treatment or intercurrent causes. As will be seen in the following chapters, contemporary palliation of these symptoms is a sophisticated art which has advanced considerably in recent years. This art is not widely taught and is therefore not routinely practised.

Three basic principles apply to the control of all symptoms: the first is to diagnose the cause, which can be multifactorial and highly complex; the second is to provide appropriate treatment; the third is to review the situation regularly in order to assess the efficacy of the treatment relative to the changing circumstances of the patient. Control of symptoms is an end in itself whatever the stage of the disease.

Unfortunately, many doctors and nurses (and even patients) accept some symptoms as inevitable, and insufficient attention is given to their control. Patients with advancing cancer may well be chronically anxious and depressed with due cause, but such symptoms can be anticipated and helped by a positive and sensitive attitude to individual needs. The recent rapid growth of the British Association of Cancer United Patients (BACUP) is evidence that many patients find it difficult to obtain information about their disease and treatment, and have to seek help from others because their individual needs are not being met.

It is a common and erroneous belief that pain relief at an early stage will inevitably lead to uncontrollable pain at the end (Twycross and Wald, 1976). A patient with a local recurrence of rectal carcinoma may have pain such that he is unable to sit down, yet if no distant spread has been identified, he may live for several years. If active treatments with radiotherapy, nerve block etc. have failed and morphine is the only drug which will control his pain, then this should be prescribed—at regular intervals, by mouth and at a dose titrated to his particular requirements. Failure to do this will condemn him to a life of poor quality. As his disease progresses he may well need an increasing dose, but tolerance is not a problem that need concern the patient. Neither is addiction a problem, and if the pain is relieved by some other means, then even high doses of morphine can gradually be discontinued completely over a period of a few days.

Other common myths are that radiotherapy always causes nausea and vomiting, and that cytotoxic chemotherapy always causes nausea, vomiting and hair loss. Radiotherapy, especially at palliative dosage, rarely causes nausea and vomiting unless the irradiated volume includes the upper lumbar region or very large fields are used (as in hemi-body radiotherapy). By no means all cytotoxic drugs cause nausea and vomiting, and recent advances have been made by oncologists in the control of these symptoms. Only a minority of cytotoxic drugs cause hair loss, and scalp cooling immediately before and after an injection can prevent hair loss in the case of some drugs (Dean et al, 1979).

A precise understanding of the aetiology of symptoms and the mode of action of different therapies is fundamental to the management of symptoms. There are, however, other factors which influence therapeutic decisions and these include an assessment of the unwanted side-effects of the treatment, the effect of the treatment on prognosis, and, not least, the wishes of the patient. Decisions can be enormously difficult, and warrant discussion with others concerned with the management of the patient and with the family. For example, active intervention may prolong life but may or may not be the best decision for an individual patient. This applies to the irradiation of cerebral metastases which are causing mental confusion in a patient with advanced bronchial carcinoma, or the insertion of ureteric catheters in a patient with symptoms of uraemia due to ureteric obstruction by an advanced carcinoma of the cervix.

Similarly nasogastric and parenteral feeding may be the only way to maintain adequate nutrition and hydration and yet may be inappropriate at the end of life for a patient who wishes to die at home, especially as there are other methods of controlling the associated symptoms as described in later chapters. Patients and families can be included in the making of these difficult decisions, but the doctor should make it quite clear that it is he who carries ultimate responsibility and accountability, in order to relieve them from this burden.

PALLIATIVE RADIOTHERAPY, CHEMOTHERAPY AND SURGERY

Radiotherapy, chemotherapy and surgery play an important role in palliative cancer management, even in the terminal phase. Here they are being used outside clinical trials in circumstances when the benefits of treatment for the patient clearly outweigh the disadvantages. In the main, the aim of such active but palliative treatment is to relieve distressing symptoms, rather than to prevent symptoms which may never arise or to prolong life. There are of course exceptions, and on some occasions all three aims may be achieved. The skill of the oncologist is manifested in knowing when to start, stop and reintroduce such treatment.

It is not always easy to refuse treatment to a patient. Very often the oncologist has known the patient for years and has helped him in the past, and both the patient and his relatives may beg for help once again. In addition, he may be pressed to treat a patient by his medical colleagues, who themselves have nothing more to offer but wish to give some positive help. On the other hand, it may happen that an oncologist who feels he can help a patient may be faced by medical or (more often) nursing colleagues, who seek to protect a patient from further therapeutic interference.

In all cases, the physician must be clear in his own mind what he can hope to achieve by his therapy. Although he will take psychological factors into consideration, he must be motivated by the possible physical benefit to his patient. Occasionally a radiotherapist may be asked to 'pretend to treat' a patient, but such deception is never justified and indeed is not necessary in the context of a team approach to palliative cancer care.

Palliative radiotherapy, if it is available, is particularly valuable. Many symptoms such as cancer pain, bleeding and offensive fungation can be relieved, often completely, by a short, low dose course of radiotherapy with few or no associated side-effects (Bates, 1984). Severe pain due to bone secondaries can often be relieved in a single treatment (Price et al, 1986).

About 40% of all cancer patients receive radiotherapy at some stage in their disease (Cohen et al, 1982), and about half the workload of a modern radiotherapy department is concerned with palliative treatment. Effective treatment requires a full range of radiotherapy equipment to deal with tumours at different depths and sites and an organization which permits treatment without delay. Radiotherapy equipment is expensive and there is much to be said for centralization of equipment, although it may be preferable to decentralize pre-treatment and follow-up care (Meredith, 1968). Ideally, travelling should be kept to a minimum, but if patients have to travel long distances for treatment, hostel beds are often appropriate and are less expensive than hospital beds.

Palliative chemotherapy may involve treatment with hormone modulating or cytotoxic drugs. Hormone therapy is generally less toxic than cytotoxic therapy but only approximately 30% of all cancers of the breast, prostate and endometrium show response to such treatment. Some cytotoxic drugs give rise to unpleasant side effects (a variable degree of nausea and vomiting, hair loss or bone marrow depression, etc.) and some can be hazardous to the user during their preparation if inhaled or spilt on the skin. It is therefore essential that their prescription and preparation are under the control of a cancer team experienced in their use. Cytotoxic drugs are most effective in the lymphomas and to a lesser extent in the treatment of solid tumours: in particular, cancers of the testis, breast, ovary and small cell carcinoma of the bronchus, and in many tumours arising in children.

Because cytotoxic chemotherapy is a relatively new and rapidly developing form of treatment, many patients receive this treatment in the context of a clinical trial. It is essential in such trials that the assessment of a patient's response to treatment should include not only an accurate record of tumour response but also a measure of side-effects and their effect on the quality of the patient's life. There is a current tendency to over-treat with chemotherapy outside clinical trials merely as a demonstration of 'we never stop trying'. This is inappropriate treatment and it must not be overlooked that many of these drugs are expensive. A survey in the USA suggests that 17% of cancer patients currently receive cytotoxic chemotherapy (DeVita, 1983) and in most of these patients, it is given in the knowledge that cure is not possible.

Palliative surgery includes the internal fixation of pathological fractures;

the relief of intestinal and urinary obstruction and spinal cord compression; the removal of large tumour masses prior to chemotherapy; endocrine ablative procedures for patients with hormone-sensitive tumours, and the resection of solitary lung or liver metastases. Surgeons may be less than enthusiastic about operating on patients who cannot be cured and who have a very short life expectancy, especially if inadequate funding limits the number of their beds and their operating time. They (and those who fund them) need to be reminded of the dramatic relief of pain which follows surgical fixation of pathological fractures, and the crucial preservation of mobility and sphincter control which follow prompt surgical relief of early spinal cord compression.

ALTERNATIVE MEDICINE

When conventional medicine fails to provide adequate palliative care, 'alternative medicine' often appears attractive. Low protein or macrobiotic diets, coffee enemas, carrot juice, vitamins and bio-feedback, meditation and faith-healing all have their vogue. While they may give considerable help to patients in terms of psychological support and comfort, there is no scientific evidence that they are of value in controlling the cancer. A possible danger is that they may be used exclusively, and thereby deprive a patient of useful conventional treatment.

PALLIATIVE CARE FOR THE TERMINAL CANCER PATIENT

Over the last 25 years the rapid growth of the British Hospice Movement has brought with it a new awareness of what can be achieved by good palliative cancer care. Hospice medicine is emphasized in this chapter because it has provided an important means of teaching the new skills and changing attitudes to treatment which are stressed in this book.

Some 134 270 patients die of cancer each year in England and Wales: 60% die in an 'acute hospital', 30% at home and a small minority in special hospices for the dying (OPCS, 1984). Most patients want to die at home and many more of them could do this if their symptoms were better controlled and if their families had more support. Beds in 'acute hospitals' are expensive and because priority is given to those patients who can be cured, it is often difficult to satisfy the particular problems of dying patients and their distressed families. One aim of good palliative cancer care is to help patients to spend as much time as possible at home and to die at home if that is their wish.

Special facilities for the terminally ill cancer patient include:

- in-patient hospice units (sometimes known as Palliative Care Units or Continuing Care Units),
- home care teams,
- hospital support teams,
- day-care centres.

No one of these facilities is necessarily better than the others. Together they form a comprehensive service aimed to meet the varied needs of patients and families. Planners need to look at what each has to offer in relation to local needs and the finance available, and to plan closely with neighbouring districts to minimize the cost of a comprehensive provision (King's Fund and NAHA, 1987).

Hospices

Some in-patient hospice units in the UK are free-standing, others are part of a general hospital. A hospice unit differs from a nursing home or a general hospital ward in that it is staffed by doctors and nurses who have had special training in terminal care. It should have a high nurse–patient ratio (at least 1.3:1) so that the staff have the time to give high quality palliative care. It should be visited regularly by oncologists and also by specialists in nerve block techniques, so that the full range of palliative care is available. It is important that hospices have strong ties with mainstream medicine so that they do not become isolated and so that they can act as a focus of expertise, research and training in palliative medicine. This experience will then extend outside the hospice for the benefit of cancer patients with a longer prognosis.

A common economic size for a hospice is 25 beds. The number of hospice in-patient units in the UK has risen rapidly, largely in response to public demand and without a co-ordinated plan, from 11 in 1960 to 109 in 1987 (Table 2). The current need is thought to be 40–50 beds per million

Table 2. Hospice care in the UK.

	1960	1970	1980	1983	1987
In-patient units	11	17	55	77	109
Home care teams (community based)	—	1	23	40	100
Hospital support teams	—	—	5	12	20
Day-care centres	—	—	1	6	53

population (Lunt and Hillier, 1981) and this figure has not yet been reached. Most of the existing units were established with charitable monies but at present the National Health Service funds 11 units built on NHS grounds, and has a contractual arrangement to fund some of the total running cost (average 38.8%) of the free-standing independent hospices. In future, it is likely that there will be closer liaison between the NHS and the charitable sector and this should result in improved monitoring and a more controlled expansion. The long-term need is for a limited number of high quality units, their precise number depending on training and service needs.

Home care teams

Many hospices have a home care team of nurses who help to look after patients in their own home, often extending care into the pre-terminal phase. They supplement the care that is already available from the family doctor, the community nurses and the social services. These teams do not take over the community nurse's role but act in an advisory and supportive manner at the invitation of the family doctor. They are often available 24 hours a day, 7 days a week. There are in the UK 100 home care teams based in the community, with others hospital- or hospice-based. They usually comprise two to six specially trained nurses with community experience. Ideally, they are backed up by a doctor skilled in palliative care. The total number of home care teams in the UK has risen from one in 1970 to 170 in 1987.

Hospital support teams

An extension of the hospice concept has been the establishment of a hospice team in acute general hospitals. The first of these teams in the UK, known as the 'Support Team', was set up at St Thomas' Hospital in London in 1977 (Bates et al, 1981). This team works both in the hospital and in the surrounding community, and its aim has been to improve the standard of care of patients with incurable cancer and to teach the skills of terminal care. Early referral, a year or more before death, is encouraged.

The St Thomas' Hospital team comprises four specialist nurses, a medical social worker, an occupational therapist, a secretary and a full-time experienced hospice doctor, plus the hospital chaplain. The team acts in an advisory capacity and has no designated hospice beds. Patients are referred to the team by their hospital consultant or family doctor and the subsequent care of the patient is shared. In this way a large number of doctors and nurses learn hospice skills. At any one time the team is caring for approximately 15–20 in-patients and 40 out-patients.

There are now 20 hospital support teams in the UK, and many are in the planning stage. They vary in size and composition; some have grown out of a pain relief clinic, some are part of the oncology department and some have designated beds. It would not be unreasonable to recommend that a support team be established in every large district general hospital. Good management and a clear operational policy are crucial to the success of such teams as they must work in parallel with so many other services both in the hospital and in the community.

Day-care

There are 53 day-care centres in the UK in 1987 where patients go by day and later return home. They give the patient a 'day out' and a change of scene and also permit more detailed medical care than is possible at home. Day-care can relieve family strain and sometimes enables a spouse to continue in employment. In economic terms, day-care helps patients to remain at home and is highly cost effective in releasing hospital and hospice beds.

TRAINING IN PALLIATIVE CARE

The current generation of doctors has had very little teaching in palliative and terminal care. Until relatively recently, specific teaching in subjects such as care of the dying, communication skills and the control of severe chronic cancer pain and other distressing symptoms were not included in the syllabus for undergraduates (or indeed, that for training of cancer specialists). Future change can therefore only be slow because of the shortage of knowledgeable teachers. The impetus to train doctors in these skills has come largely, though not entirely, from those practising hospice medicine, and the problem is compounded because hospice doctors in the UK have no recognized career structure and none of their few training posts carry formal accreditation.

Clearly there is a need for medical education in palliative care at two levels: first, basic education for all at undergraduate and postgraduate level; second, specialist education, with long- and short-term accredited training posts, for those wishing to specialize full-time in palliative medicine and also for family doctors and oncologists.

Basic education in palliative cancer care should be part of the teaching course both in general oncology and general practice. Medical students are particularly receptive to the subject at the end of the pre-clinical course when many medical schools hold an introductory clinical course. Integrated teaching throughout the clinical course will be reinforced by the possibility of a question in examinations. At postgraduate level, it is the junior doctors who are the most receptive as they carry the responsibility for the day to day management of patients, not least for the control of their distressing symptoms. Experience with the St Thomas' Hospital Support Team suggests that more effective teaching can be achieved by the regular presence of the team on busy wards than by formal lectures, and that more teaching can be done in general wards than in separate palliative care beds where care is not shared. All teaching hospitals would benefit from a well-run multidisciplinary palliative care team on the premises, and all major cancer centres should have access to such services for both in- and out-patients.

Specialist education in these skills will inevitably be limited until there is a recognized career structure for hospice doctors in the UK, and approved posts for higher training in palliative care for those entering general practice and oncology. However, encouraging signs are the increasing number of courses, symposia and conferences on aspects of palliative cancer care for all disciplines, and the increasing interest in the subject shown in medical and nursing literature.

SUMMARY

Many cancer patients, even in the most prestigious cancer centres in the UK, suffer unnecessarily. Many oncologists, because of deficiencies in their education, find it difficult to focus on the patient's quality of life, and give a great deal more emphasis to length of survival and to measurements of temporary tumour response to treatment. Symptom control is no less important and is fundamental to good management. The high quality of palliative care described in hospice literature should be routinely available to cancer patients throughout the palliative phase, and not reserved just for those who are acknowledged to be dying.

Attitudes are changing and there is a growing interest in palliation, not as a 'soft option' but as a sophisticated skill. As this skill requires more time than is generally available to a busy doctor, a closer interaction between doctor and nurse is developing, with nurses and others extending the care previously given by the doctor. Other valuable developments are the growth of cancer support services and patients' self-help groups.

At the end of the day, it is the clinician who makes therapeutic decisions as the agent of the patient, and co-ordinates the hopes of the patient and relatives with the realities of the situation. In this aim he selects treatment compassionately, and personally takes responsibility for controlling distressing symptoms whether due to disease or to treatment. It is hoped that this book will help him in such care.

REFERENCES

Bates TD, Hoy AM, Clarke DG & Laird PP (1981) The St Thomas' Hospital Terminal Care Support Team—A New Concept of Hospice Care. *Lancet* **i:** 1201–1203.

Bates TD (1984) Radiotherapy in Terminal Care. In Saunders CM (ed.) *The Management of Terminal Disease*, pp 133–138. London: Edward Arnold.

Brinkley D & Haybittle JL (1977) The Curability of Breast Cancer. *World Journal of Surgery* **1:** 287–289.

Cancer Statistics Registry, England and Wales (1986) Series B1 No. 15. London: Her Majesty's Stationery Office.

Cohen SS, Connolly CC, Matthews GC & Skeet R (1982) Information Needs for Radiotherapy Services. *British Journal of Radiology* (British Institute of Radiotherapy Bulletin) **55:** B51–B54.

Dean JC, Salmon MD & Griffiths RN (1979) Prevention of Doxorubicin-induced Hair Loss with Scalp Hypothermia. *New England Journal of Medicine* **301:** 1427–1432.

DeVita VT (1983) Progress in Cancer Management. *Cancer* **51:** 2401–3409.

Haybittle JL (1983) What is Cure in Cancer? In Stoll BA (ed.) *Cancer Treatment, Endpoint Evaluation*, pp 3–21. Chichester: John Wiley.

King Edward's Hospital Fund for London and National Association of Health Authorities (1987) *Care of the Dying. A Guide for Health Authorities.* Birmingham: NAHA.

Lunt B & Hillier R (1981) Terminal Care: Present Services and Future Priorities. *British Medical Journal* **283:** 595–598.

Meredith JW (1968) What Manchester thinks . . . (The Sylvannus Thompson Memorial Lecture). *British Journal of Radiology* **41:** 2–11.

Office of Population Censuses and Surveys (1984) Mortality Statistics for 1983 England and Wales, Series DH1 No. 9. London: Her Majesty's Stationery Office.

Price P, Hoskin PJ, Easton D, Austin D, Palmer SG & Yarnold JR (1986) Prospective randomised trial of single and multifraction radiotherapy schedules in the treatment of painful bony metastases. *Radiotherapy and Oncology* **6:** 247–255.

Saunders CM (1984) *The Management of Terminal Disease.* London: Edward Arnold.

Soukop M & Calman KC (1977) Cancer Patients: Where do They Die—An Analysis. *Practitioner* **219:** 883–888.

Twycross RG & Wald SS (1976) The Long Term Use of Diamorphine in Advanced Cancer. In Bonica JJ & Albe-Faascard D (eds) *Advances in Pain Research*, Volume 1. pp 653–661. New York: Raven Press.

Twycross RG & Lack SA (1983) *Symptom Control in Far Advanced Cancer: Pain Relief.* London: Pitman.
Twycross RG & Lack SA (1986) *Control of Alimentary Symptoms in Far Advanced Cancer.* Edinburgh: Churchill Livingstone.
Waterhouse JAH (1974) *Cancer Handbook of Epidemiology and Prognosis.* Edinburgh-London: Churchill Livingstone.

2

Dyspnoea

A. M. HOY

Dyspnoea is common in patients dying of cancer. Figures from both St Christopher's and St Joseph's Hospices in London show that approximately half of all patients complain of breathlessness on admission to these institutions. The percentage is higher for men, reflecting the greater incidence of bronchial tumours (Haram 1984, Heyse-Moore 1984). As a cause of suffering it ranks with unrelieved pain, yet in many ways it is less easy to palliate.

Dyspnoea is defined as difficulty in breathing. In the context of palliative care for the cancer patient, this difficulty implies both the perception of the sensation of breathlessness but also the subjective reaction to that sensation. Breathlessness caused by the physical exertion of a normal person running upstairs may be quantitatively similar to that of a cancer patient walking on level ground. However, the cancer patient is likely to perceive his breathlessness as more distressing than that of the normal person because it may cause anxiety by underlining the presence of progressive disease. The study of dyspnoea as with pain must allow for the subjectiveness of the patient's reaction to increased respiratory effort. Although increased respiratory rate (tachypnoea) and depth (hyperpnoea) may not necessarily be distressing to all cancer patients, the definition of dyspnoea must be wide enough to cover tachypnoea and hyperpnoea. Dyspnoea results when there is either increased ventilatory demand or decreased ventilatory capacity. In cancer patients both these factors may be present simultaneously, e.g. a patient with fever (increased demand) and pleural effusion (decreased capacity). It is necessary to consider physiological and pathological aspects of dyspnoea in order to understand appropriate palliative measures.

PHYSIOLOGY

Breathing is under dual control: (1) automatic control mediated via the brain stem and (2) voluntary modification of breathing initiated as a conscious act via the cerebral cortex, thus allowing breath holding, talking and singing.

Ventilation is achieved by the motor activity of the diaphragm and the intercostal muscles. These are directly controlled by anterior horn cells of C3-5 and T1-12 segments of the spinal cord respectively. Increased ventilatory demand will result in the use of the accessory respiratory muscles such as sternomastoid. This is precipitated in normal subjects by vigorous exercise, but in dyspnoeic patients may occur at rest. In automatic breathing, the anterior horn cells of the spinal cord are controlled by the medullary respiratory complex (MRC), whereas voluntary control is exercised directly via the cerebral cortex. The MRC is influenced by both chemical and neurogenic stimuli. Chemical stimuli include hypoxaemia, hypercapnia and other causes of acidaemia such as uraemia, diabetes mellitus or salicylate toxicity. Hypoxaemia is sensed principally by peripheral arterial chemoreceptors and relayed via the glossopharyngeal nerve. Hypercapnia is detected by central medullary chemoreceptors situated close to the MRC. Neurogenic stimuli include proprioceptor input from the respiratory muscles, mechanoreceptor information from the larger airways and the lung parenchyma, intrapulmonary irritant receptors and juxtacapillary (J) receptors. These last three types of receptor all transmit information via the vagus nerve. More central neurogenic influences on the MRC come from ascending spinal pathways and from the reticular formation. It is likely that information from joint and muscle receptors in moving limbs contributes to this stimulatory spinal influence on the MRC. Finally the information which comes from the γ system of the muscle spindles within the respiratory muscles is thought to be important in the appreciation of unusually large respiratory efforts producing dyspnoea. The control of respiration is summarized in Figure 1.

MECHANISM OF DYSPNOEA

Although it might seem easy to assess the mechanism of dyspnoea in

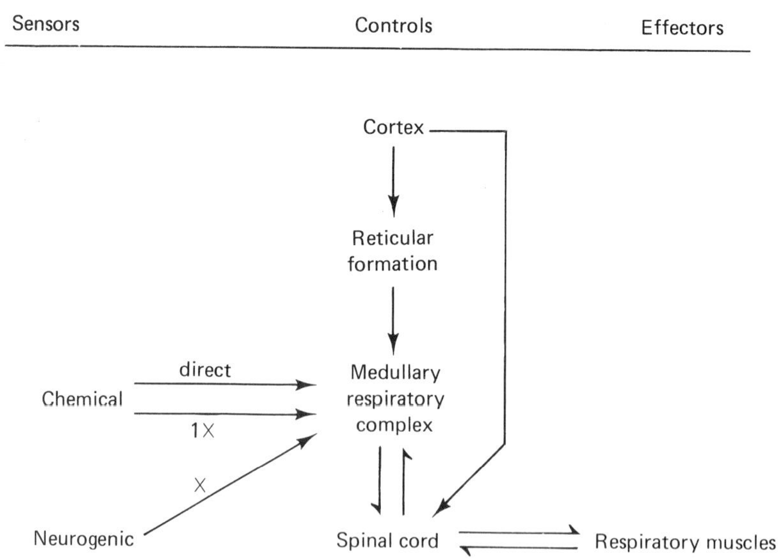

Figure 1. Control of respiration.

individual patients with disordered physiology, in practice this is not the case. The origin of the unpleasant sensation of breathlessness remains an enigma (Anon 1986). Degrees of dyspnoea due to disease can be quantified relatively consistently by various techniques such as visual analogue scales, but the use of artificially induced hypoxia or hypercapnia to stimulate ventilation experimentally produces responses that differ widely depending on mood and other psychological or social factors. Campbell and Howell (1963) proposed the hypothesis of 'length–tension inappropriateness' of respiratory muscle as being the primary factor in the perception of dyspnoea. This is the degree of lung expansion achieved in relation to the force required. This hypothesis has been supported by clinical observation (Leblanc et al 1986) but it is difficult to separate cause from effect.

There is speculation as to which of the respiratory sensors mediate feelings of dyspnoea. As regards the intrapulmonary sensors, stretch receptors are concerned with the Hering-Breuer reflex which is no longer thought to be important in adult man unless tidal volume exceeds one litre (West 1985); irritant or rapidly adapting receptors are concerned with dyspnoea only if it is caused by inhalation of noxious substances or bronchoconstriction associated with histamine release. The J receptors closely related to pulmonary capillaries within the alveolar wall have been implicated as mediating dyspnoea in various pathologies (Paintal 1977). Although interruption of the vagus was useful for some causes of dyspnoea (Guz et al 1970) inactivation of J receptors by inhalation of fine particle local anaesthetic has not however proved useful for dyspnoea in chronic lung disease (Stark et al 1985).

What about the arterial chemoreceptors being the pathway through which dyspnoea is appreciated? Studies involving first chemically stimulated dyspnoea and then 'voluntary copying' of the previously observed reflexly produced respiratory excursions demonstrate that both the stimulus and the response must be present before there is a conscious perception of dyspnoea (Adams et al 1985). This agrees with the observation that dyspnoea is not perceived following C3 cord transection.

In summary, the mechanism of dyspnoea is 'the perception of a reflexly mediated need for increased ventilation' which requires the integrity of both afferent and efferent pathways to the respiratory muscles. Palliation must depend on decreasing the need for ventilation or alteration of the unpleasant perception.

AETIOLOGY

Dyspnoea in terminal malignant disease has various causes. These are summarized in Table 1. They include pulmonary, neuromuscular, cardiovascular, metabolic and psychogenic causes. Several may be operating simultaneously in the often complex clinical situation found in these patients. Dyspnoea is frequently accompanied by hypoxaemia, and indeed this is the most common sensory stimulus in the 'dyspnoeic reflex'. However, hypoxaemia is not invariably present. Causes of dyspnoea which increase the ventilatory demand such as anxiety, fever or acidosis do so by

Table 1. Causes of dyspnoea in terminal malignant disease.

Pulmonary	*Cardiovascular*
Obstructive	Ischaemia
Restrictive	Embolism
V/Q inequality	Tamponade
Loss of surface area for diffusion	Arrhythmia
Alveolar–capillary block	Anaemia
Hypodynamic	*Metabolic*
Neuromuscular	Diabetes mellitus
Generalized weakness	Uraemia
Chest wall pain	Salicylates
Tetraplegia	Pyrexia
Diaphragmatic splinting	*Psychogenic*

means other than hypoxaemia. Pulmonary and neuromuscular causes imply inadequate ventilation. The cardiovascular causes include both pump failure but also inadequate oxygen carrying capacity of the blood.

Pulmonary

Obstruction of the airways may occur anywhere throughout the respiratory tract. Tumour may cause dyspnoea in the nose, pharynx, larynx, trachea and bronchi. Upper airway obstruction is often associated with other symptoms such as nasal discharge, dysphagia or hoarseness. The obstruction may be intrinsic or extrinsic such as compression of the airway by thyroid tumour, or neck and mediastinal lymphadenopathy. The obstruction may also be functional in the case of vocal cord paralysis. This is commonly caused by compression of the left recurrent laryngeal nerve by tumour at the left pulmonary hilum, but it may also be due to neck metastases or direct laryngeal invasion. Laryngeal stridor may also be caused by oedema due to superior vena caval obstruction.

Intraluminal obstruction may be caused by blood, vomit, pus or retained mucus. This is common distal to a stenotic bronchial tumour and may lead to segmental or whole lung consolidation and collapse. Aspiration of saliva and food occurs with oesophageal obstructions, causing overflow. Occasionally a tracheo-oesophageal fistula develops because of tumour invasion and necrosis. In this case acute dyspnoea is precipitated by swallowing and drinks are immediately expectorated.

Finally many patients have coexisting obstructive airways disease either of long standing or they may develop bronchospasm associated with their terminal illness.

Restrictive defects of lung function cause dyspnoea by reducing the total lung capacity. The lung compliance (the volume change produced by a given distending pressure) is reduced. The lung has become stiffer. This occurs when there is diffuse interstitial intrapulmonary tumour, lymphangitis carcinomatosa, or when multiple areas of lung are involved with discrete metastases. Compliance is also reduced by pulmonary oedema due to congestive cardiac failure or fluid from pneumonia and by fibrosis due to either

either disease or radiotherapy. Restrictive defects may also be due to extrapulmonary factors which prevent adequate ventilation such as pleural effusions or tumour.

Ventilation/perfusion (V/Q) inequality causes hypoxaemia either because there are ventilatory defects which are unmatched by a reduction in perfusion, or because there is overperfusion without the ability to increase ventilation and so oxygenate the blood (right to left shunt). Inequality of V/Q is present in chronic bronchitis, emphysema, multiple emboli, pneumonia, asthma and pulmonary fibrosis.

Loss of surface area for diffusion results in hypoxaemia because respiratory reserve is reduced. Dyspnoea is usually exertional but if there is considerable loss of lung tissue it will occur on talking or at rest. This is seen with emphysema, pulmonary infarction, pulmonary fibrosis, and extensive lung resection.

Alveolar-capillary block has much the same effect except that the lung tissue that is present is inefficient as a gas exchange organ. This is a feature of pulmonary oedema, asbestosis, diffuse fibrosis and lymphangitis carcinomatosa.

Hypodynamic ventilation results in hypoxaemia in chronic bronchitis, severe asthma and extreme obesity.

Neuromuscular

Many terminally ill dyspnoeic patients are frail and cachectic. They are often bed bound for reasons other than their dyspnoea and they may occasionally have non-metastatic neuropathy or myopathy which contributes to neuromuscular hypoventilation. Painful chest wall or rib tumours will act as a restrictive ventilatory defect. If muscular weakness is very severe the conditions for 'length–tension inappropriateness' are not satisfied and dyspnoea is not a problem. However, weak and cachectic patients commonly become dyspnoeic terminally if only by virtue of difficulty in expectorating intraluminal secretions. This 'death rattle' may be distressing to both patient and onlooker and should be regarded and treated as a special case of dyspnoea.

One or other of the two respiratory effectors, the intercostal muscles or the diaphragm may be inactive and so contribute to inadequate ventilation. This occurs when a patient is either tetraplegic due to low cervical cord compression, or has diaphragmatic splinting due to ascites or hepatomegaly.

Cardiovascular

When dyspnoea has a cardiac cause, pulmonary oedema results in hypoxaemia because of alveolar capillary block. There is often pulmonary disease present which may have caused cor pulmonale and the hypoxaemia itself will exacerbate myocardial failure. Ischaemic heart disease is common generally and often contributes to failure, as does anaemia. Thromboembolism is common in cancer patients and may have been the presenting feature of a malignancy. Carcinomas of the bronchus may invade the pericardium causing effusion or cardiac arrhythmias. Tamponade due to pericardial effusion presents with severe dyspnoea often with rapid onset. Arrhythmias may cause palpitations, dizziness, sweating and sometimes angina if they are severe enough to cause dyspnoea. The arrhythmias may be paroxysmal or continuous.

Metabolic

Tachypnoea and hyperventilation due to uraemia or diabetic ketoacidosis may be severe enough to cause complaint. However, there are likely to be other features which contribute to the clinical picture such as polydipsia and polyuria, or vomiting. Any diabetic tendency may have been exacerbated by corticosteroid treatment. Large doses of salicylates may also cause hyperventilation. Many patients with terminal malignancy have overt infections either of the respiratory tract or elsewhere. This may give rise to pyrexia, tachycardia and tachypnoea.

Psychogenic

Anxiety can be a potent cause of dyspnoea either alone or as part of a vicious circle of breathlessness. Pure psychogenic dyspnoea is often described in terms of being 'suffocating', or 'not able to take a complete breath' in spite of the absence of any particular distress. Organic causes of dyspnoea must be excluded although patients may be quite willing to acknowledge and discuss the 'panic' element of their symptoms.

DIFFERENTIAL DIAGNOSIS

Symptom relief, just like accurate diagnosis, requires skilful clinical assessment. The quality, timing, severity and circumstances of the dyspnoea must be determined. Descriptions of dyspnoea may include 'wheezing' or 'blowing' in obstructive airways disease, or an experienced chest clinic patient may comment on new or different features; however, qualitative terms are generally less useful for dyspnoea than for symptoms such as pain.

Timing and speed of onset may be much more helpful. Sudden onset dyspnoea over a period of minutes suggests a cardiovascular cause such as embolism, arrhythmia or acute left ventricular failure. Onset over hours or days will include pneumonia, asthma, pleural or pericardial effusions, metabolic and some neuromuscular causes. Onset over weeks or months will suggest increasing tumour growth, fibrosis, weakness, multiple small emboli and anaemia.

Objective evidence of the severity of dyspnoea must be assessed. Performance of daily tasks such as dressing, walking, climbing stairs or even just talking will often give useful comparative information from day to day.

Circumstances which precipitate or exacerbate dyspnoea will often give useful clues to the cause. Orthopnoea, paroxysmal nocturnal dyspnoea and frothy sputum are suggestive of left ventricular failure. Accompanying palpitations or anginal pain may indicate paroxysmal arrhythmia. Patients with asthma may be able to identify specific precipitating factors such as house-dust mite, animal danders, exercise, cold air inhalation or fumes. A history of dyspnoea only at rest and not on exertion suggests a psychogenic cause.

Clinical assessment includes inspection of the sputum. Infection is common and may be a treatable cause of diminished respiratory reserve. A history of night sweats, haemoptysis, weight loss, corticosteroid administration and radiotherapy may all be consistent with bronchial carcinoma but examination and culture of the sputum may also reveal acid fast bacilli.

Physical examination will indicate the degree of systemic distress of the patient. The presence of cyanosis indicates severe hypoxaemia but this will be absent if there is significant anaemia; conversely, secondary polycythaemia of chronic respiratory disease will cause cyanosis without severe hypoxaemia. The cyanosis must be central (lips, tongue and conjunctivae) to be significant as peripheral cyanosis occurs normally with cold extremities or any degree of circulatory shut down. Respiratory rate, use of accessory muscles and intercostal recession may be useful as comparative indices. However, respiratory rate itself may be inconsistent unless assessed unobserved or while the patient is asleep. Patients with chronic obstructive disease have a hyperinflated barrel chest often with very limited respiratory excursion. Differential chest expansion between the two sides is a useful sign. It may indicate pleural effusion, consolidation, collapse or fibrosis on the side of diminished movement. Superior vena caval obstruction is obvious clinically with the presence of dilated neck and arm veins and conjunctival oedema. However, it should be remembered that the more florid the chest wall veins appear, the more chronic the obstruction will be and therefore there will be less urgency for treatment and less response anticipated.

Palpation and percussion may indicate tracheal and cardiac displacement suggesting unilateral pleural effusion, pneumothorax, collapse or fibrosis. Rib tenderness will indicate bony metastases or cough fracture both of which produce a restrictive pattern of dyspnoea. Abdominal examination may reveal hepatomegaly or ascites which may be restricting expansion by splinting the diaphragm. Shoulder tip pain on deep inspiration may indicate diaphragmatic irritation due to hepatic or splenic infarction.

Cardiovascular assessment will include signs of right or left heart failure. Low blood pressure, pulsus paradoxus, raised jugular venous pressure and inaudible heart sounds are suggestive of tamponade. An arrhythmia such as fast atrial fibrillation may be obvious clinically or it may be necessary to confirm the diagnosis with an electrocardiogram. Sudden onset dyspnoea caused by massive pulmonary embolism is often accompanied by crushing chest pain, hypotension, cyanosis and a gallop rhythm. Acute left ventricular failure may be caused by myocardial infarction or decompensated aortic or mitral valve disease. Sometimes dyspnoea due to pulmonary oedema can be associated with wheezing which may make the differential diagnosis more difficult.

Auscultation of the lungs may be confounded in the terminally ill by severe cachexia, shivering, or if the patient is too ill to be moved about in bed. Absent or reduced breath sounds indicate lack of air entry to the underlying lung although if consolidation is present the large airway noises are transmitted producing bronchial breathing. An exception to this finding is when there is consolidation beneath a pleural effusion. Breath sounds are usually absent in this situation, probably because the combination of fluid and collapsed lung is a poor sound conductor. Similarly vocal resonance and fremitus are increased in the presence of lung consolidation, but voice transmission is reduced over an effusion. On occasion a bleating quality (aegophony) is heard above the level of the effusion.

Added sounds are either crackles (crepitations), wheezes (rhonchi) or a rub. Fine crackles sound like hair being rubbed between fingers and indeed a hairy-chested patient may have artefactual fine crackles. Their presence at the lung bases indicate pulmonary oedema. Coarse crackles are heard in various clinical situations including normal individuals. They may change after coughing, but in terminally ill patients they usually indicate intraluminal secretion or interstitial fibrosis. Wheezes or rhonchi indicate partial obstruction in the lumen of bronchi. If they are inspiratory and fixed they indicate large airway obstruction by tumour. If they are higher pitched, widespread and expiratory they indicate bronchitis or asthma. Expiratory wheezes in terminally ill dyspnoeic patients always suggest the possibility of symptomatic relief with bronchodilators. A rub has a creaking sound and is caused by two roughened serous surfaces moving against each other. The rub is heard over the area of pleura involved, both during inspiration and then at the equivalent phase of expiration. The underlying condition is any cause of inflammation, pleural or pericardial. This includes pleural tumour, infection, pulmonary embolism and occasionally hepatic irritation of the diaphragm. An audible pleural rub will often coincide with the patient complaining of pleuritic pain. If a sizeable pleural effusion develops the pleural rub will disappear as the two adjacent surfaces are separated.

Clinical assessment alone will often indicate the cause of dyspnoea in terminally ill patients, however confirmatory investigations may be helpful. These include chest X-ray, ECG, sputum culture, blood gas estimation, routine blood count and clinical chemistry. Lung function tests and V/Q scans are occasionally helpful, although most clinicians would think twice before advising anticoagulation for pulmonary embolism in terminally ill patients.

MANAGEMENT

Relief of dyspnoea can be obtained by treatment of the cause if that is at all possible. If the specific cause is untreatable, as is often the case, then it is necessary to alter the 'perception of the reflexly mediated need for ventilation' by reducing respiratory drive centrally. This can be achieved with small doses of any respiratory depressant, but regular opioids will also reduce anxiety and relieve discomfort if this is implicated in dyspnoea as with chest wall pain. Oral morphine 2.5–5 mg four hourly is usually sufficient yet does not depress the MRC enough to cause measurable increase in $P\text{CO}_2$ (Heyse-Moore 1984).

Pulmonary causes

Infection underlies many pulmonary causes of dyspnoea. Unless tuberculosis is suspected empirical use of a broad spectrum antibiotic is more sensible than awaiting the questionable result of sputum culture and sensitivities. Oral amoxycillin, erythromycin or cotrimoxazole for up to seven days is the treatment of choice. The use of antibiotics for palliation of dyspnoea demands an assessment of how effective they are likely to be but also whether temporary resuscitation is really in the patient's best interests. Aggressive treatment of infection may merely prolong a patient's life for a relatively short and distressing period. It is often possible to obtain a clear idea of the views and wishes of both patient and family. Conversely, a few days of even symptomatic life may be exactly what a patient requires, possibly for family, social or financial reasons. Symptom control must therefore take account of social as well as physical distress.

Obstructive airways disease whether acute or chronic may have elements of reversibility which will relieve dyspnoea. Bronchodilator therapy may increase a patient's respiratory reserve just enough to relieve their dyspnoea. As time is often short, a reasoned polypharmaceutical approach is recommended. A selective β_2-adrenoceptor stimulant such as salbutamol or terbutaline combined with the atropine-like effect of ipratropium should be given four hourly. If the patient is unable to use an inhaler then a compressed air nebulizer is efficient and effective. However, a nebulizer must be used only under supervision. This usually implies inpatient treatment only. Doses are salbutamol 2.5 mg and ipratropium 250 micrograms given over 10–15 minutes. Nebulizers are capable of delivering much higher doses than inhalers and therein lies advantage and hazard. Dose reduction may be required if problems are caused by excessive tremor, tachycardia or, rarely, angina. An oral xanthine derivative such as aminophylline, if given as a sustained release preparation, may be helpful particularly for nocturnal wheezing. Aminophylline (Phyllocontin Continus) 225 mg increasing to 450 mg twice daily can be added to nebulizer therapy. Finally a corticosteroid (dexamethasone 8 mg/day) should be added. As well as its bronchodilatory action it may also reduce peri-tumour oedema and ease dyspnoea in lymphangitis carcinomatosa. This bronchodilator/steroid regime may be more effective with the addition of a diuretic if there is a possibility of pulmonary oedema. As long as two weeks may be required before symptomatic improvement is evident in the presence of chronic airways obstruction and extensive pulmonary tumour.

Restrictive defects of lung function may respond to both corticosteroids and diuretics as above, but extrinsic factors such as pleural effusion or ascites may be equally important. An active approach is worth considering as development of malignant pleural effusion does not necessarily imply a short prognosis. Median survivals of 6–16 months have been quoted depending on the primary tumour (Dhillon and Spiro 1983). Simple aspiration will give symptomatic relief but the fluid usually reaccumulates within 3 days. Successful pleurodesis depends on complete drainage and therefore apposition of parietal and visceral pleural surfaces, and an effective sclerosing agent which will remain within the pleural space without systemic side-effects. The various sclerosing agents have been compared, with talc poudrage giving the best control rate of 90% (Fentiman et al 1986). The disadvantages of using talc are that a general anaesthetic is required, which may be hazardous, experienced operator and anaesthetist are essential, and selection of the relatively long prognosis patients who would benefit is not always easy (Fentiman, 1987). Drainage and instillation of quinacrine or tetracycline with lignocaine is a better although rather less effective option in patients who are more ill. There is little evidence that the use of intracavity cytotoxics or radionuclides have any advantage over simple sclerosants.

Paracentesis for abdominal ascites is effective in relieving dyspnoea but similar problems of reaccumulation occur. Sclerosing agents are rather less successful than with pleural fluid. If the patient has a relatively long prognosis then insertion of a peritoneo–venous shunt should be considered. LeVeen or Denver shunts can be inserted under sedation and local anaesthesia. Venous access is obtained via a jugular vein. Complications include clotting of the shunt in the presence of bloody or high protein content ascites. Less clotting occurs with the Denver shunt (Mauch and Ultmann 1985).

Other pulmonary causes of dyspnoea such as V/Q inequality, loss of surface area for diffusion, alveolar–capillary block and hypodynamic ventilation are often due to irreversible structural pathology and offer only limited opportunity for intervention. Pulmonary oedema, pneumonia and embolism may be treatable but it may not always be appropriate to do so aggressively. Hypoxaemia can be corrected partially by breathing oxygen. This often relieves dyspnoea in the short term, but the difficulties of long term continuous domiciliary supply, the hazards of suppression of anoxic drive in chronic bronchitics, the inevitable dry mouth, and cylinder dependence mean it is best avoided if possible.

Specific oncological treatments such as radiotherapy, chemotherapy and hormone therapy may be useful in the relief of dyspnoea. A recently obstructed large bronchus will often open up following palliative radiotherapy, or suitable chemotherapy if the tumour is chemo-sensitive. As a longer term treatment, a hormone manipulation in the presence of a hormone-sensitive tumour may ease symptoms due to parenchymal disease or pleural effusion.

Physiotherapy is useful for retained secretions, to help with postural drainage of partially blocked bronchi, breathing exercise retraining and relaxation. However, inappropriate enthusiasm must be avoided in view of the possibility of rib metastases.

Neuromuscular causes

Of the neuromuscular causes of dyspnoea, chest wall pain is relatively easy to relieve. Conventional regular analgesia may be all that is required but palliative radiotherapy for pathological rib fracture or vertebral metastases may be useful. Single doses of 8 Gy to the ribs or short courses of 20 Gy in five daily fractions are usually well tolerated and effective (Hoy 1984). Nerve blocking procedures are particularly helpful in relieving chest wall pain. Intercostal block, if necessary of multiple segments, can be carried out with bupivacaine as a bedside procedure. If this is successful a more permanent block should be used with phenol or cryoprobe (Bonica 1984). Paravertebral block may be required if the pain is spinal in origin.

Cardiovascular causes

For the cardiovascular causes of dyspnoea various specific treatments are useful. Conventional diuretics will reduce pulmonary oedema due to ischaemic congestive failure. Anticoagulation may be life prolonging in the presence of thrombo-embolic disease. Pericardial aspiration often improves severe dyspnoea due to tamponade. However, this procedure should be carried out only under appropriate ECG control with the availability of resuscitation equipment. Recurrent pericardial effusion in an otherwise fit patient may require pericardial window formation as an open operation. This allows dispersal of any fluid into the much larger pleural space. Accurate characterization of cardiac arrhythmias is important for treatment. Fast atrial fibrillation or flutter is often symptomatic and digoxin is the treatment of choice. Blockade of β-adrenoceptors or verapamil may be necessary for persistent supraventricular tachycardia. However, caution is required as hypotension, cardiac failure and asthma can be precipitated. Cardioselective β-blockers such as atenolol are less likely to cause asthma. Finally, dyspnoea due to anaemia often responds to transfusion. Patients may be elderly and therefore fluid overload and pulmonary oedema is always a possibility.

Metabolic causes

Metabolic causes of dyspnoea should be treated if possible. Diabetes may be steroid induced and this is usually easy to control by reducing steroid dose and giving glibenclamide according to blood sugar readings or urinalysis. Uraemia will often be due to obstructive uropathy from recurrent pelvic malignancy. Not only will this be difficult to treat but it may not be appropriate inasmuch as death from renal failure may be a relatively peaceful end.

Psychogenic causes

Anxiety is frequently a component of dyspnoea whatever other pathology may be present. The use of low dose opioids has been mentioned. Addition of a small dose of diazepam (2–5 mg) eight hourly is often very helpful without causing undue sedation or respiratory depression. Techniques of relaxation, deep breathing and retraining have been mentioned and are often valuable for psychogenic dyspnoea.

Death rattle

Terminally, bronchopneumonia, retained secretions and aspiration of saliva can usually be dried up by regular hyoscine or atropine. If a patient is stuporose and unable to swallow, a syringe containing diamorphine 10 mg (or more if pain is a problem), hyoscine 2.4 mg and haloperidol 10 mg given subcutaneously by a syringe driver over 24 hours will ease terminal dyspnoea.

PROGNOSTIC SIGNIFICANCE

The causes of dyspnoea are so varied that it is difficult to attach prognostic significance to dyspnoea in general. However, the major precipitants of death in cancer patients are infection and organ failure (Hoy 1987). Pneumonia has been termed 'the old man's friend' and dyspnoea due to infection has a particular serious significance. Recent onset cyanosis implies progressive hypoxaemia given a normal haemoglobin. This is usually of significance. Some other causes of dyspnoea such as coexisting chronic obstructive airways disease may be compatible with relatively long life expectation. Dyspnoea due to cachexia and the various cardiovascular causes must clearly imply a short prognosis.

REFERENCES

Adams L, Lane R, Shea SA et al (1985) Breathlessness during different forms of ventilatory stimulation: a study of mechanisms in normal subjects and respiratory patients. *Clinical Science* **69:** 663–672.

Anonymous (1986) The enigma of breathlessness. *Lancet* i: 891–892.

Bonica JJ (1984) Local anaesthesia and regional blocks. In Wall PD, Melzack R (eds) *Textbook of pain*, pp 541–557. Edinburgh: Churchill Livingstone.

Campbell EJM & Howell JBL (1963) The sensation of breathlessness. *British Medical Bulletin* **19:** 36–40.

Dhillon DP & Spiro SG (1983) Malignant pleural effusions. *British Journal of Hospital Medicine* **29:** 506–510.

Fentiman IS (1987) Effective treatment of malignant pleural effusions. *British Journal of Hospital Medicine* **37:** 421–428.

Fentiman IS, Rubens RD & Hayward JL (1986) A comparison of intracavity talc and tetracycline for the control of pleural effusions secondary to breast cancer. *European Journal of Cancer and Clinical Oncology* **22:** 1079–1081.

Guz A, Noble NIM, Eisele JH, et al (1970) Experimental results of vagal block in cardiopulmonary disease. In Porter R (ed) *Breathing: Hering–Breuer centenary symposium* pp 315–328.

Haram BJ (1984) Facts and Figures. In Saunders C (ed) *The management of terminal malignant disease*, pp 13–16. London: Edward Arnold.

Heyse-Moore L (1984) Dyspnoea. In Saunders C (ed) *The management of terminal malignant disease*, pp 113–119. London: Edward Arnold.

Hoy AM (1984) Radiotherapy, chemotherapy and hormone therapy: treatment for pain. In Wall PD, Melzack R (eds) *Textbook of pain*, pp 753–764. Edinburgh: Churchill Livingstone.

Hoy AM (1987) Clinical pointers to prognosis in terminal disease. In Stoll BA (ed) *Pointers to cancer prognosis*, pp 79–88. Dordrecht: Martinus Nijhoff.

Leblanc P, Bowie DM, Summers E, et al (1986) Breathlessness and exercise in patients with respiratory disease. *American Reviews of Respiratory Diseases* **133:** 21–25.

Mauch PM & Ultmann JE (1985) Treatment of malignant ascites. In DeVita VT, Hellman S, Rosenberg SA (eds) *Cancer principles and practice of oncology*, pp 2150–2153. Philadelphia: Lippincott.

Paintal AS (1977) Thoracic receptors concerned with sensation. *British Medical Bulletin* **33:** 169–174.

Stark RD, O'Neill PA, Russell NJW, et al (1985) Effects of small particle aerosols of local anaesthesia on dyspnoea in patients with respiratory disease. *Clinical Science* **69:** 29–36.

West JB (1985) Control of ventilation. In West JB (ed) *Best and Taylor's physiological basis of medical practice*, pp 605–613. Baltimore: Williams and Wilkins.

3

Anorexia and cachexia

KENNETH C. H. FEARON
KENNETH C. CALMAN

The majority of patients with malignant disease lose weight (Nixon et al, 1980) and a proportion become emaciated to the extent that they appear to die of starvation (Warren, 1932; Inagaki et al, 1974). This syndrome is known as cancer cachexia. The term cachexia is derived from the Greek words kakos meaning bad and hexis meaning condition. Patients with cancer cachexia are characterized by the presence of anorexia, early satiety, severe weight loss, weakness, anaemia and oedema (Calman, 1982). The importance of gross cachexia as a major factor contributing to the morbidity and mortality of cancer patients is clearly established (Warren, 1932). However, recent data also point to an association between minor weight loss and a shortened duration of survival. Indeed, the prognostic effect of weight loss may be greatest in patients with a more favourable prognosis i.e. good performance status or limited tumour spread (DeWys, 1986). This suggests a very subtle relationship between nutritional status and the outcome of malignant disease.

Weight loss does not correlate with the type of cancer, the duration of the disease or with the site or number of metastases (Costa and Donaldson, 1979). However, the incidence is greatest with gastro-intestinal and lung tumours (Strain, 1979). Where a tumour is associated with the gastro-intestinal tract it might be expected to affect appetite, digestion and absorption with a resulting state of malnutrition (Lawrence, 1979). How similar effects can be caused by a tumour in the lung is more difficult to explain.

In spite of a vast literature on the subject the mechanisms by which tumours produce the symptoms of cachexia remain unknown (Schein et al, 1974) and this is due largely to a lack of systemic studies of the problem. The techniques available for use in human studies are severely limited by ethical considerations and it is only recently that suitable animal models of cachexia have become available (Coombes, 1982). Despite substantial interindividual variation, patient studies have been carried out on small numbers and often the results are not generally applicable. Furthermore, many of the patients have already undergone some form of therapy or are at different stages in the development of cachexia. Comparisons between studies is, therefore, often impossible and the literature is replete with confusing and contradictory results.

In general, loss or gain of body mass is due to an imbalance between energy intake and expenditure. The aim of much clinical research has been to determine whether it is an increased energy expenditure, a reduced food intake, or a combination of the two that leads to weight loss in the majority of cancer patients. Numerous studies have documented abnormalities of host metabolism which together indicate that cancer cachexia is not the same as simple starvation (Brennan, 1977). It is the aim of this chapter to discuss the factors which might contribute either to anorexia or abnormal host metabolism and to examine the best clinical methods of overcoming the anorexia–cachexia syndrome.

This chapter is divided into two sections. The first section deals with mechanisms and management of anorexia in cancer patients. Particular emphasis is given to treatment of symptoms which might contribute to anorexia and to methods of maintaining an adequate oral intake. The second section details the metabolic problems which may contribute to the development of cachexia and discusses the indications for nutritional intervention in patients with malignant disease.

ANOREXIA

Anorexia is a frequent and often demanding symptom in patients with cancer (DeWys, 1979). Patients complain of a loss of appetite and a tendency to feel 'full' after ingesting only a small amount of food. As many as 40% of patients attending a standard oncology outpatient clinic will complain of loss of appetite (Willox et al, 1984). Appetite may be defined as that set of signals which guide the selection and consumption of specific foods and nutrients (Castonguay et al, 1983). Anorexia occurs, therefore, when these signals are absent or abnormal, causing the individual to lose the desire for food or specific food stuffs. In the very extensive literature on the subject over the last 50 years, there has been a tendency to look for a single mechanism by which appetite could be controlled. Over this time, however, it has become clear that a multiplicity of mechanisms is involved. In a similar fashion, the search for a unifying mechanism of anorexia in patients with cancer has revealed a very complex situation indeed.

Numerous clinical factors can be easily identified which may contribute to the development of anorexia in cancer patients. These include intestinal obstruction, radiotherapy- or chemotherapy-induced nausea and vomiting, altered taste sensitivity, oral ulceration, depression and anxiety. However, some patients can be profoundly anorectic for no identifiable physical or psychological reason. In this group, reference to postulated normal mechanisms of appetite control has revealed several possible mechanisms of anorexia and numerous potential methods for therapeutic intervention.

Under normal circumstances appetite is thought to be regulated both by long-term and short-term feedback systems. A long-term feedback is suggested by the fact that individuals tend to maintain their body weight and composition over very long periods despite markedly changing circumstances (Brobeck, 1960; Mayer et al, 1954). A short-term feedback system is suggested by the fact that an individual usually becomes hungry, starts eating and stops eating from meal to meal.

The signals involved in the long-term feedback system are unclear. Nevertheless, it is evident that the hypothalamus acts as the integration centre. For example, Anand and Brobeck (1951) recorded that animals with centromedial hypothalamic lesions increased their food intake so that an increased but stable body weight was reached. This has led to suggestions of a 'set-point' mechanism within the hypothalamus. The presence of this 'set-point' has, however, been disputed recently (Morley and Levine, 1983).

Numerous signals have been perceived to act in the short-term control of appetite. These include changes in blood glucose, free fatty acid or amino acid concentrations, altered neuronal activity as a result of distension of the gastro-intestinal tract or alterations in the concentrations of various hormones such as insulin, glucagon, bombesin or cholecystokinin (Von Meyenfeldt and Soeters, 1986). Alterations in blood glucose, free fatty acid and amino acid kinetics have all been documented in cancer patients (Wesdorp, 1986) and it is possible that these changes contribute to the development of anorexia with weight loss. Moreover, it is clear that abnormal neuronal or hormonal signals from the gastro-intestinal tract might arise as a result of involvement by the malignant process and thus contribute to anorexia.

It has also been proposed that decreased binding of tryptophan to albumin in the cancer host might increase the precursor pool for cerebral serotonin synthesis (Krause et al, 1979). Increased serotonin turnover has been correlated with the onset of anorexia in rodent models of cancer cachexia (Von Meyenfeldt et al, 1982). Thus, abnormal host metabolism might directly influence neurotransmitter concentrations in the hypothalamic appetite centres. However, the precise role of any of these potential mechanisms of anorexia in cancer patients remains to be defined.

Management of anorexia and reduced food intake

There are several approaches to the management of anorexia in cancer patients, including treatment of contributing factors, modification of feeding pattern and the use of appetite stimulants and oral nutritional supplements. The use of fine bore nasogastric feeding and parenteral nutrition is discussed later.

Factors which contribute to anorexia and which may be effectively dealt with include taste abnormalities, pain, nausea, constipation and oral ulceration or infection. Patients who complain that food has lost its taste may have an elevated threshold for sweetness and may benefit from increased seasoning or flavouring of their food (DeWys, 1977). Patients often complain that they are no longer able to eat or enjoy red meat. Advice to try fish or poultry may be helpful. Alternatively, eggs, cheese, milk or pulses can act as an adequate protein source.

Pain can often interfere with patients' ability to perform the normal activities of daily living. Adequate pain control throughout the day, but especially at meal times, may lead to a substantial improvement in oral intake. Some may suffer from severe nausea, either as a result of metastatic disease (especially hepatic metastasis) or because of recent radiotherapy or chemotherapy. Even if vomiting is not a problem, it is most important to control nausea with frequent and regular doses of standard anti-emetics. Depression, anxiety and stress can all interfere with food intake. Emotional supportive care and provision of adequate community resources can help alleviate such problems.

Oral ulceration or infection can markedly reduce a patient's voluntary food intake. Oral hygiene is often neglected whether the patient is at home or in hospital. Ill-fitting dentures and dental caries may contribute to oral infection. Moreover, chemotherapy and radiotherapy can cause severe oral ulceration and the debilitated cancer patient who is immunosuppressed, and has poor saliva production, is liable to develop oral candidiasis (Samaranayake et al, 1984). These problems can be overcome with frequent antiseptic mouth washes, nystatin for oral candidiasis and acyclovir to arrest progression of herpes simplex.

The principles of behaviour modification therapy can be used to encourage an increased oral food intake (DeWys and Herbst, 1977). This involves educating the patient; establishing a limited and potentially achievable target of food intake; and measuring and providing regular feedback. Because regaining lost weight is often unachievable, the goal best suggested is maintenance of current weight. Body weight is measured at regular visits to the out-patient clinic and patients are given feedback on the basis of the result.

Early satiety is a problem which describes patients who are unable to tolerate or consume the volume of food required to maintain body weight. This may be due to previous upper gastro-intestinal surgery (e.g. partial gastrectomy) but most commonly the cause is unknown. Milk-based oral food supplements of high calorie and protein value offer one way of overcoming this problem. There are numerous commercial products currently available (e.g. Buildup, Complan). These products often taste rather bland or even unpleasant. However, some savoury flavours are now available and altering the texture of these supplements by cooling or mixing with other food is often helpful in maintaining a patient's interest.

The aim of such supplemental feeding should be to provide adequate energy and protein for patients to maintain their body weight and if possible return to their normal body composition. For the average sedentary individual a maintenance regimen might require 1500–2000 kcal and 45–75 g of protein. Most supplemental feeds contain 1 kcal/ml. Thus, an individual who is managing to eat two-thirds of his dietary requirement would only need to ingest approximately 500 ml of supplement to attain a positive energy and protein balance.

Finally, it is most important to remember that the help of a dietitian in the out-patient care of patients with cancer can be invaluable. Such an individual may help with the assessment of a patient's nutritional status, instruct patients how to eat a balanced diet, provide suggestions on methods of overcoming problems with taste, sore mouth, etc., and advise on the use of oral supplements. In addition, the oncology dietitian provides a further line of communication and source of information as part of the multidisciplinary team approach to cancer medicine.

In addition to these general measures various pharmacological agents have been used in the management of anorexia in cancer patients.

Hormones

Anabolic hormones, usually testosterone derivatives, have been widely used (Freuhan and Frawley, 1963). They have a small effect on weight gain and appetite stimulation. Moreover, some studies have shown a reduction in weight loss sustained during intensive chemotherapy if an anabolic steroid is given at the same time (Chlebowski et al, 1982). Prednisolone in small doses has been shown to stimulate appetite. Willox and co-workers (1984) demonstrated in a double blind placebo controlled trial that 5 mg of prednisolone three times a day gave significant improvement though this was short lived.

Drugs acting on the central nervous system

These drugs have been used because of their interaction with the neurotransmitters in the hypothalamus. Of the phenothiazines, haloperidol (1 mg twice a day) relieved nausea, vomiting and anorexia in patients receiving chemotherapy (Cole and Duffy, 1974). Of the antidepressants, amitriptyline hydrochloride may increase the appetite acting as a serotonin antagonist. The cannabinoid derivatives (Sallan et al, 1975) in addition to having anti-emetic effects may also increase appetite.

Other compounds

Various other compounds with appetite stimulant properties have been tried in patients with cancer cachexia. Cyproheptadine hydrochloride, a serotonin antagonist has been shown to be of limited value (Irsy and Szatloczky, 1977). Hydrazine sulphate, a compound known to inhibit gluconeogenesis, has also been shown to have significantly greater appetite stimulant properties than a placebo (Chlebowski et al, 1985). Of general interest is the use of high doses of vitamin C which, whilst having no effect on survival, did seem to increase well-being and appetite over short periods of time (Creagen et al, 1979). Alcohol is a well known appetite stimulant, when used in moderation!

CACHEXIA

Anorexia and a reduced food intake undoubtedly contribute to the severe wasting observed in most patients with cancer cachexia. Nevertheless, it has been shown that cancer cachexia is not the same as simple starvation (Brennan, 1977). Thus it has been proposed that there must be a metabolic component contributing to weight loss in some, if not all, cancer patients. In order to understand and therefore treat the metabolic aspects of cancer cachexia it is necessary first to understand both the normal mechanism of energy balance in the body and the changes involved during adaptation to starvation.

Starvation and the metabolism of the cachectic cancer host

The body requires energy and this is obtained either from food or from body fuel stores. During a prolonged period without food the energy and amino acids which are normally provided by the diet have to be obtained by the breakdown of body tissues and it is this process which leads to the emaciation characteristic of starvation. Fat is the major energy reserve in the body and loss of adipose tissue during starvation is well tolerated. However, there is no specific store of protein in the body and daily amino acid requirements have to be met by the breakdown of structural and functional proteins. Clearly vital organs such as the heart need to be preserved for as long as possible. Therefore, during prolonged starvation the body first mobilizes protein from low priority tissues such as skeletal muscle. Thus the tissues most affected by starvation are adipose tissue and skeletal muscle. However, the selectivity of wasting is not absolute and visceral protein is also lost.

One factor which contributes to protein loss in early starvation is the inability of the brain to use free fatty acids as substrate for energy production. Glucose is the preferred fuel and this is obtained by the release of amino acids from skeletal muscle which are then converted into glucose by the liver and kidney (Owen et al, 1969). Thus during early starvation the body excretes about 12 g of nitrogen per day principally as a result of muscle proteolysis. If this process continued unabated the duration of survival would be limited due to a rapid loss of lean tissue. However, in response to starvation ketone bodies are generated in the liver from free fatty acids and these replace glucose as the main substrates for cerebral energy metabolism (Robinson and Williamson, 1980). Thus the need for amino acids for gluconeogenesis is greatly reduced, the rate of muscle proteolysis is decreased, and the rate of nitrogen excretion in compensated starvation is only about 2 g of nitrogen per day (Cahill, 1970).

This ordered pattern of metabolic adaptation would appear to be disrupted by the presence of the tumour. Various alterations of carbohydrate, protein and fat metabolism have been described in cancer patients. Those most likely to contribute to weight loss are described below.

Carbohydrate metabolism

In contrast with compensated starvation the rate of gluconeogenesis from alanine (Waterhouse et al, 1979), lactate (Waterhouse, 1974; Holroyde et al, 1975) and glycerol (Lundholm et al, 1982) has been shown to be increased in various groups of cancer patients. The mechanism of this accelerated gluconeogenesis is not clearly established. In 1930 Warburg observed that tumours metabolize glucose via glycolysis at a high rate, whilst in normal cells this pathway is usually reserved for anaerobic conditions. Subsequently, several studies demonstrated a high rate of glycolysis in tumours and a dependence on glucose as an energy source (Gold, 1966; Shapot and Blinov, 1974; Demetrakopoulos et al, 1978). Gold (1968) proposed that this high glucose demand by the tumour is an important factor in the development of cachexia. He suggested that body fat and protein reserves are depleted in order to provide substrates for gluconeogenesis. The glucose so produced is metabolized by the tumour which releases lactate into the bloodstream. The lactate is then transported to the host's liver where it is converted back to glucose. The cycle from glucose to lactate and back to glucose is known as the Cori cycle and a 2–3-fold increase in the activity of this cycle has been reported in cachectic cancer patients (Waterhouse, 1974). Since the anaerobic breakdown of glucose to lactic acid yields only two molecules of ATP and the resynthesis of glucose from lactate requires six molecules of ATP, this cycle is very wasteful of energy compared with the potential 36 molecules of ATP via the aerobic oxidation of glucose. However, since cachexia can develop in the presence of a very small tumour burden (Costa, 1977) and since some tumours that produce cachexia do not have increased rates of glycolysis (Weinhouse, 1982) the suggestion that cachexia is caused by the high glucose demand of the tumour does not seem generally applicable.

Protein metabolism

Protein metabolism in the tumour bearing host also appears to be different from that of uncomplicated starvation. Lundholm and co-workers (1976) demonstrated a decreased rate of protein synthesis and an increased rate of protein degradation in muscle biopsies from cachectic cancer patients. This observation would account for a net protein mobilization. Moreover, the reduced protein synthesis rate is consistent with the pattern observed in starvation (McNurlan et al, 1980). However, in contrast to the overall depletion of muscle protein, a marked increase in liver mass accompanies the growth of several tumours (Stewart and Begg, 1953; Lundholm et al, 1979; Heymsfield and McManus, 1985). Unlike the changes observed in starvation, the liver seems to be protected from the net negative nitrogen balance in the tumour bearing host such that an increased rate of hepatic protein synthesis has been described (Lundholm et al, 1979; Emery et al, 1984). An increased rate of protein synthesis in the liver and a decreased rate in skeletal muscle, together with the additional protein synthesis occurring in the tumour, is thought to result in an apparently normal to increased rate of protein synthesis and turnover in the whole body (Jeevanandam et al, 1984; Eden et al, 1984). This is in sharp contrast to the decreased rates of whole body protein turnover and synthesis observed during uncomplicated starvation (Rennie et al, 1982).

Fat metabolism

Fat metabolism in the cancer-bearing host is also abnormal. Fat is mobilized as the major energy reserve during starvation; the free fatty acids released are oxidized to provide energy and the glycerol backbone is converted to glucose via gluconeogenesis. Administration of glucose during starvation reduces both free fatty acid oxidation and gluconeogenesis and it is thought that this effect is mediated by insulin (Butcher, 1968). In contrast, free fatty acid oxidation continues in the presence of administered glucose in cachectic cancer patients (Waterhouse and Kemperman, 1971).

Although these observations support the suggestion that cancer cachexia may not be entirely consistent with semi-starvation the question remains as to which metabolic abnormalities are significant and how they induce weight loss.

Mechanisms of weight loss in cancer

In order to determine possible mechanisms of weight loss in cancer patients it is necessary to consider the factors which keep the body weight stable in normal individuals. When the energy lost as mechanical work or as heat is balanced by the energy obtained from food in the diet the body weight remains stable. Therefore, loss or gain of body mass is due to an imbalance between energy intake and energy expenditure. A number of studies have looked for an imbalance in this relationship in cachexia. Walsh and co-workers (1983) and Cohn and colleagues (1981) both demonstrated a marked reduction of food intake in cancer patients who had become severely cachectic. However, in contrast, when cancer patients were studied during the early phase of weight loss a reduction in food intake was not observed (Costa et al, 1981).

Whether or not food intake is reduced, an increased energy expenditure might account for the rapid weight loss and other symptoms of cachexia in cancer patients. Numerous investigators have used indirect calorimetry to determine whether the resting energy expenditure of patients with cancer is elevated. Lindmark and co-workers (1984) and Macfie and colleagues (1982) both demonstrated that the resting energy expenditure of patients with disseminated malignancy is increased by 5–20% when compared with controls. In contrast, Hansell and co-workers (1986) showed that there was no difference between the resting energy expenditure of large groups of patients with either lung, colon or gastric cancer and that of non-cancer controls. In another study (Dempsey et al, 1984) it was shown that approximately one-third of cancer patients were hypermetabolic, one-third were normal and one-third were hypometabolic. However, even a 'normal' rate of energy expenditure would be inappropriate in the semi-starving cancer host since the normal adaptive response to a reduction in energy intake is a decrease in energy expenditure.

The mechanisms whereby the energy expenditure of some cancer patients is increased or at least fails to adapt to the semi-starving state are unknown. One proposal is that energy dependent metabolic cycles such as protein turnover or the glucose–lactate cycle (Cori cycle) are increased. However, the relation between these abnormalities and the metabolic rate, increased or otherwise, is not clear. Although some investigators have found a correlation between an increased Cori cycle activity and weight loss (Holroyde et al, 1975), other workers have failed to do so (Kokal et al, 1983). Similarly, whole body protein turnover has been shown to be elevated in some groups of malnourished cancer patients (Jeevanandam et al, 1984; Eden et al, 1984) but not in others (Glass et al, 1983). Thus, as yet, it is unclear whether the weight loss of cancer patients is primarily due to a reduced food intake, an increased energy expenditure or a combination of the two. Moreover, the mechanism of any proposed elevation of energy expenditure is not established.

The reasons for abnormalities of protein, fat, carbohydrate and energy metabolism which have been documented in the cancer host are unknown. Indeed, it is not even clear if the observed changes form a consistent pattern such that all cases of cancer cachexia can be classed as a single syndrome. Cachexia can arise in humans when a tumour is less than 0.01% of host weight (Morrison, 1976) yet some patients with very large tumours show no sign of cachexia (Stein, 1978). Thus, it is unlikely that the metabolic demands of the tumour constitute a significant drain on host metabolism. An alternative theory is that tumours produce small-molecular weight peptides which are capable of altering the activity of various host enzymes. Because this occurs in a random manner, a state of metabolic chaos is produced (Theologides, 1977). However, although human tumours are known to be capable of both exocrine (Coombes, 1982) and autocrine (Sporn and Todaro, 1980) secretion of polypeptides, no tumour-specific product has yet been shown to be responsible for the metabolic defects which are thought to contribute to cachexia.

It has also been suggested that some of the metabolic abnormalities in cancer cachexia are similar to those observed in trauma and sepsis (Brennan, 1977). The loss of body fat and protein in patients with trauma or sepsis is thought to result from a combination of altered hormone profiles superimposed on semi-starvation (Wilmore, 1983). Many of the metabolic events of trauma or sepsis (e.g. hyperglycaemia, increased nitrogen loss) can be reproduced by a combined infusion of glucagon, cortisol (hydrocortisone) and adrenaline (Bessey et al, 1984). However, several aspects such as fever and production of acute phase proteins are not observed following such an infusion. The latter phenomena may be due to peptide lymphokines (e.g. interleukin-1 and tumour necrosis factor) which are produced by inflammatory cells in response to injury and infection (Dinarello, 1985). Moreover, these mediators may enhance net triglyceride mobilization from adipose tissue (Beutler et al, 1985a,b) and amino acid release from skeletal muscle (Baracos et al, 1983). Thus the inflammatory response and the release of these mediators may be a key component in the events leading to body wasting associated with disease. In humans with cancer, tumour necrosis, destruction of normal tissue and infection are just some of the factors independent of tumour type that could elicit such an inflammatory response. The hypothesis that the metabolic abnormalities observed in cancer cachexia are due to mediators of the inflammatory response remains to be examined in detail.

Treatment of cancer cachexia

Clearly, the best way to resolve the nutritional and metabolic abnormalities resulting from the growth of a tumour is the removal of the tumour (Calman, 1982). However for the majority of solid epithelial malignancies, once the tumour has spread beyond the organ of origin, chemotherapy, radiotherapy or surgery will not effect a cure and may even worsen the nutritional deficit of the patient (Ohnuma and Holland, 1977; Kokal, 1985). Thus, whilst the search continues for more effective antineoplastic therapy, attention has been focused on supportive measures to reduce the morbidity and mortality which result from the nutritional problems associated with progressive tumour growth (Copeland et al, 1977).

With the advent of fine-bore nasogastric feeding and safe total parenteral nutrition the past decade has seen intensive investigation of the role of nutritional support in cancer patients. The aims of such support have fallen into two broad areas: (1) reversal of the cachectic state with relief of associated symptoms; (2) the improvement of host tolerance to chemotherapy, radiotherapy or surgery. It is now clear that nutritional supplementation is not the panacea it promised to be. Nevertheless, the achievements of this era have been to place the role of nutritional supplementation in proper perspective and to outline new areas for future investigation.

Efficacy and limitations of nutritional supplementation

Because it is cheap, safe and has distinct metabolic advantages over the parenteral route, enteral hyperalimentation is the method of choice where a functional gastro-intestinal tract is present. Enteral hyperalimentation can be either through the use of oral supplements in the form of high protein/calorie drinks (e.g. Complan, Buildup) or by the infusion of similar products (e.g. Ensure) through a fine-bore nasogastric tube. Alternatively, the parenteral route may need to be used, especially in the depleted patient receiving aggressive antineoplastic therapy where nausea and vomiting may preclude use of the gastro-intestinal tract. An added advantage of providing nutritional supplementation by either nasogastric feeding or parenteral hyperalimentation is that they both obviate the problem of anorexia and early satiety.

Methods of central venous cannulation and metabolic monitoring for parenteral hyperalimentation are beyond the scope of this chapter and are described in detail elsewhere (Fearon and Calman, 1986). However, in general, the aim of supplementation would be to administer about 50% more energy and amino acids than the patient's basal requirements. Thus, in order to promote a positive energy and nitrogen balance a typical regimen might contain 2500 kcal and 14 g nitrogen.

Numerous studies have been performed to determine the response of the cancer host to nutritional supplementation. Unfortunately, it is now clear that not all the aims of such supplementation can be realized. The metabolism of the cancer bearing host is not consistent with that of compensated semi-starvation (Brennan, 1977) and similarly the response to nutritional supplementation would appear to be less than that which can be achieved in the malnourished patient with chronic benign disease (Nixon et al, 1981a). If weight gain can be achieved, fat deposition occurs more readily than repletion of the vital lean body mass (Cohn et al, 1982). The nature of this partial block to the repletion of host lean body mass remains unknown, though clearly it is related to the continued growth and activity of the patient's neoplasm. Nevertheless, despite often ineffective antineoplastic therapy, it must be emphasized that even the arrest of weight loss or a small gain in weight can accompany a much greater improvement in functional activity and psychological well-being in the wasted cancer patient given nutritional supplementation.

Interaction of nutritional support and antineoplastic therapy

Both enteral and parenteral hyperalimentation have been tested extensively as adjuncts to surgery, radiotherapy and chemotherapy. Within this context, nutritional support has been given either to allow already severely malnourished cancer patients to receive aggressive antineoplastic therapy or to try and prevent the catabolic sequelae of such management. Furthermore, animal studies suggesting that the response to chemotherapy could be improved and tolerance to chemotherapy increased by concomitant total parenteral nutrition (Steiger et al, 1975; Cameron and Rogers, 1977; Souchon et al, 1975) led to trials assessing such effects in patients.

In the first instance, non-randomized studies suggested an improved response to chemotherapy when depleted cancer patients were given concurrently, parenteral nutrition (Lanzotti et al, 1975; Schwartz et al, 1971). In contrast, prospective studies over a wide range of malignancies have failed to show an improved tolerance (i.e. a reduction in gastro-intestinal upset, myelosuppression or sepsis) or an increased response to chemotherapy in those randomized to parenteral hyperalimentation as opposed to voluntary oral intake (Nixon et al, 1981b; Samuels et al, 1981; Popp et al, 1981). Survival, likewise, has not been improved. Similar results have been obtained with radiotherapy (Valerio et al, 1978; Bothe et al, 1979). Several studies have, however, demonstrated improved or preserved nutritional parameters in those given total parenteral nutrition during the administration of chemotherapy (Russel et al, 1984; Valdivesio et al, 1981). Postoperative complications following surgery for upper gastro-intestinal malignancy can be reduced by a period of pre-operative hyperalimentation (Heatly et al, 1979; Muller et al, 1982). No improvement, however, in recurrence or survival following surgical management has been proven consistently.

SUMMARY AND CONCLUSIONS

The anorexia–cachexia syndrome continues as a very difficult problem in the management of cancer patients. Despite a vast literature, the aetiology of this syndrome is not clearly established. A reduced food intake and abnormal host metabolism are thought to be the major factors leading to cachexia. However, the extent to which either of these factors are present in any one group of patients is unknown, as too are the mechanisms whereby anorexia or abnormal host metabolism develop.

Nutritional supplementation can take the form of appetizing food, oral supplemental feeds, appetite stimulants, nasogastric feeding or total parenteral nutrition. With these techniques it is possible to improve the nutritional status and well-being of many patients. However, in terms of improved survival, randomized prospective studies have failed to demonstrate a consistent benefit from total parenteral nutrition given to patients undergoing aggressive antineoplastic therapy. In view of these results it is seldom justified to administer such intensive nutritional therapy. Thus, maintenance of cancer patients' nutritional status via an adequate oral intake is the primary aim of current nutritional intervention. Methods of attaining this goal are discussed at length in the text.

REFERENCES

Annand BK & Brobeck JR (1951) Hypothalamic control of food intake in rats and cats. *Yale Journal of Biology and Medicine* **24:** 123–140.

Baracos V, Rodeman HP, Dinarello CA & Goldberg AL (1983) Stimulation of muscle protein degradation and prostaglandin E2 release by leukocytic pyrogen: a mechanism for the increased degradation of muscle proteins during fever. *New England Journal of Medicine* **308:** 553–558.

Bessey PQ, Walters JM, Aoki TT & Wilmore DW (1984) Combined hormonal infusion stimulates the metabolic response to injury. *Annals of Surgery* **200:** 264–281.

Beutler B, Mahoney J, Le Trang N, Pekala P & Cerami A (1985a) Purification of cachectin, a lipoprotein lipase suppressing hormone secreted by endotoxin-induced RAW 264.7 cells. *Journal of Experimental Medicine* **161:** 984–995.

Beutler B, Greenwald D, Hulmes JD et al (1985b) Identity of tumour necrosis factor and the macrophage-secreted factor cachectin. *Nature* **316:** 552–554.

Bothe A, Valerio D, Biotrion BR & Blackburn GL (1979) Randomised control trial of hospital nutritional support during abdomino-pelvic radiotherapy (abstract). *Journal of Parenteral and Enteral Nutrition* **3:** 292.

Brennan MF (1977) Uncomplicated starvation versus cancer cachexia. *Cancer Research* **37:** 2359–2364.

Brobeck JR (1960) Food and temperature. *Recent Progress in Hormone Research* **16:** 439–466.

Butcher RW (1968) Role of cyclic AMP in hormone actions. *New England Journal of Medicine* **279:** 1378–1384.

Cahill GF (1970) Starvation in man. *New England Journal of Medicine* **282:** 668–675.

Calman KC (1982) Cancer cachexia. *British Journal of Hospital Medicine* **26:** 28–34.

Cameron IL & Rogers W (1977) Total intravenous hyperalimentation and hydroxyurea chemotherapy in hepatoma bearing rats. *Journal of Surgical Research* **23:** 279–288.

Castonguay TW, Applegate EA, Upton DE & Stern JS (1983). Hunger and appetite: old concepts, new distinctions. *Nutrition Reviews* **41:** 101–110.

Chlebowski RT, Herrold J, Richardson B & Black JB (1982) Effects of Deca-Durabolin in patients with advanced non small cell lung cancer. *Clinical Research* **23:** 541.

Chlebowski RT, Grosvenor M, Scrooc M et al (1985) Influence of hydrazine sulfate on food intake and weight maintenance in patients with cancer. *Proceedings of the American Society of Clinical Oncology* **4:** G1029 (abstract).

Cohn SH, Gartenhaus W, Vartsky D et al (1981) Body composition and dietary intake in neoplastic disease. *American Journal of Clinical Nutrition* **34:** 1997–2004.

Cohn HS, Vartsky D, Ashok N et al (1982) Changes in body composition of cancer patients following combined nutritional support. *Nutrition and Cancer* **4:** 107–119.

Cole DR & Duffy DF (1974) Haloperidol for radiation sickness. *New York State Journal of Medicine* **74:** 1558–1562.

Coombes RC (1982) Metabolic manifestations of cancer. *British Journal of Hospital Medicine* **26:** 21–27.
Copeland EM, Daly JM & Dudrick SJ (1977) Nutrition as an adjunct to cancer treatment in the adult. *Cancer Research* **37:** 2451–2456.
Costa G (1977) Cachexia, the metabolic component of neoplastic diseases. *Cancer Research* **37:** 2327–2335.
Costa G & Donaldson S (1979) Effects of cancer and cancer treatment on the nutrition of the host. *New England Journal of Medicine* **300:** 1471–1474.
Costa G, Bewley P, Aragon M & Siebold J (1981) Anorexia and weight loss in cancer patients. *Cancer Treatment Reports* **65** (supplement 5): 3–7.
Creagan ET, Moertel CG, O'Fallon JR et al (1979) Failure of high dose vitamin C (ascorbic acid) therapy to benefit patients with advanced cancer. *New England Journal of Medicine* **301:** 687–690.
Demetrakopoulos GE, Linn B & Amos H (1978) Rapid loss of ATP in malignant cells deprived from glucose in contrast to normal cells. *Biochemical and Biophysical Research Communications* **82:** 787–794.
Dempsy DT, Feurer ID, Knox LS, Crosby LO, Buzby GP & Mullen JL (1984) Energy expenditure in malnourished gastrointestinal cancer patients. *Cancer* **53:** 1265–1273.
DeWys WD (1977) Anorexia in cancer patients. *Cancer Research* **37:** 2354–2358.
DeWys WD (1979) Anorexia as a general effect of cancer. *Cancer* **43:** 2013–2019.
DeWys WD (1986) Weight loss and nutritional abnormalities in cancer patients: incidence, severity and significance. In Calman KC & Fearon KCH (eds) *Nutritional Support for the Cancer Patient*, pp 251–261. London: WB Saunders.
DeWys WD & Herbst SH (1977) Oral feeding in the nutritional management of the cancer patient. *Cancer Research* **37:** 2429–2431.
Dinarello CA (1985) An update on human interleukin-1 from molecular biology to clinical relevance. *Journal of Clinical Immunology* **5:** 287–297.
Eden E, Ekman L, Bennegard K, Lindmark L & Lundholm K (1984) Whole body tyrosine flux in relation to energy expenditure in weight-losing cancer patients. *Metabolism* **33:** 1020–1027.
Emery PW, Lovell L & Rennie MJ (1984) Protein synthesis measured in vivo in muscle and liver of cachectic tumor-bearing mice. *Cancer Research* **44:** 2779–2784.
Fearon KCH & Calman KC (1986) Methods of nutritional support for cancer patients. In Calman KC & Fearon KCH (eds) *Nutritional Support for the Cancer Patient*, pp 317–336. London: WB Saunders.
Freuhan AE & Frawley TF (1963) Current status of anabolic steroids. *Journal of the American Medical Association* **184:** 527–532.
Glass RE, Fern EB & Garlick PJ (1983) Whole body protein turnover before and after resection of colorectal tumours. *Clinical Science* **64:** 101–108.
Gold J (1966) Metabolic profiles in human solid tumours. A new technique for the utilization of human solid tumours in cancer research and its application to the anaerobic glycolysis of isologous benign and malignant colon tissues. *Cancer Research* **26:** 695–705.
Gold J (1968) Proposed treatment of cancer by inhibition of gluconeogenesis. *Oncology* **22:** 185–207.
Hansell DT, Davies JWL & Burns HJG (1986) The relationship between resting energy expenditure and weight loss in benign and malignant disease. *Annals of Surgery* **203:** 240–245.
Heatly RV, Williams RHP & Lewis MH (1979) Preoperative intravenous feeding—a controlled trial. *Postgraduate Medical Journal* **55:** 541–545.
Heymsfield SB & McManus CB (1985) Tissue components of weight loss in cancer patients: A new method of study and preliminary observations. *Cancer* **55:** 238–249.
Holroyde CP, Gabuzda TG, Putnam RC, Paul P & Reichard GA (1975) Altered glucose metabolism in metastatic carcinoma. *Cancer Research* **35:** 3710–3714.
Inagaki J, Rodriguez V & Bodey GP (1974) Causes of death in cancer patients. *Cancer* **33:** 568–573.
Irsy G & Szatloczky E (1977) Effect of peritol in stimulating appetite and promoting weight gain. *Therapia Hungarica* **25:** 115–121.
Jeevanandam M, Lowry SF, Horowitz GD & Brennan MF (1984) Cancer cachexia and protein metabolism. *Lancet* **i:** 1423–1426.

Kokal WA (1985) The impact of anti-tumour therapy on nutrition. *Cancer* **55:** 273–278.
Kokal WA, McCulloch A, Wright PD & Johnston IDA (1983) Glucose turnover and recycling in colorectal carcinoma. *Annals of Surgery* **198:** 146–150.
Krause R, James JH, Ziparo V & Fischer JE (1979) Brain TRP and the neoplastic anorexia–cachexia syndrome. *Cancer* **44:** 1003–1008.
Lanzotti VJ, Copeland EM, George SL, Dudrick SJ & Samuels ML (1975) Cancer chemotherapeutic response and intravenous hyperalimentation. *Cancer Chemotherapy Reports* **59:** 437–439.
Lawrence W (1979) Effects of cancer on nutrition. *Cancer* **43:** 2020–2029.
Lindmark L, Bennegard K, Eden E et al (1984) Resting energy expenditure in malnourished patients with and without cancer. *Gastroenterology* **87:** 402–408.
Lundholm K, Bylund AC, Holm T & Schersten T (1976) Skeletal muscle metabolism in patients with malignant tumour. *European Journal of Cancer* **12:** 465–471.
Lundholm K, Ekman L, Edstrom S, Karlberg I, Jargenburg R & Schersten T (1979) Protein synthesis in liver tissue under the influence of a methylcholanthrene-induced sarcoma in mice. *Cancer Research* **39:** 4657–4661.
Lundholm K, Edstrom S, Karlberg I, Ekman L & Schersten T (1982) Glucose turnover, gluconeogenesis from glycerol, and estimation of net glucose cycling in cancer patients. *Cancer* **50:** 1142–1150.
Macfie J, Burkinshaw L, Oxby C, Holmfield JHM & Hill GL (1982) The effect of gastrointestinal malignancy on resting metabolic expenditure. *British Journal of Surgery* **69:** 443–446.
Mayer JNB, Marshall JJ & Vitale JH (1954) Exercise, food intake and body weight in normal rats and genetically obese adult mice. *American Journal of Physiology* **177:** 544–548.
McNurlan MA, Pain VM & Garlick PJ (1980) Conditions that alter rates of tissue protein synthesis in vivo. *Biochemical Society Transactions* **8:** 283–285.
Morley JE & Levine AS (1983) The central control of appetite. *Lancet* **i:** 398–401.
Morrison SD (1976) Control of food intake in cancer cachexia: A challenge and a tool. *Physiology and Behaviour* **17:** 705–714.
Muller JM, Brenner U, Dienst C & Pichlmaier H (1982) Pre-operative parenteral feeding in patients with gastrointestinal carcinoma. *Lancet* **i:** 68–71.
Nixon DW, Heymsfield SB, Cohen AE et al (1980) Protein calorie under-nutrition in hospitalised cancer patients. *American Journal of Medicine* **68:** 683–690.
Nixon DW, Lawson DH, Kutner M et al (1981a) Hyperalimentation of the cancer patient with protein calorie undernutrition. *Cancer Research* **41:** 2038–2045.
Nixon DW, Moffit S, Lawson DH et al (1981b) Total parenteral hyperalimentation as an adjunct to chemotherapy of metastatic colorectal cancer. *Cancer Treatment Reports* **65** (supplement 5): 121–128.
Ohnuma T & Holland JF (1977) Nutritional consequences of cancer chemotherapy and immunotherapy. *Cancer Research* **37:** 2395–2406.
Owen OE, Felig P, Morgan AP, Wahren J & Cahill GF (1969) Liver and kidney metabolism during prolonged starvation. *Journal of Clinical Investigation* **48:** 574–583.
Popp MB, Fisher RI, Wesley R, Aamodt R & Brennan MF (1981) A prospective randomised study of adjuvant parenteral nutrition in the treatment of advanced diffuse lymphoma: influence on survival. *Surgery* **90**(2): 195–203.
Rennie MJ, Edwards RHT, Halliday D, Matthews DE, Wolman SL & Millward DJ (1982) Muscle protein synthesis measured by stable isotope techniques in man: the effects of feeding and fasting. *Clinical Science* **63:** 519–523.
Robinson AM & Williamson DH (1980) Physiological roles of ketone bodies as substrates and signals in mammalian tissues. *Physiological Reviews* **60:** 143–187.
Russel D McR, Shike M, Marlios EB et al (1984) Effects of total parenteral nutrition and chemotherapy on the metabolic derangements in small cell lung cancer. *Cancer Research* **44:** 1706–1711.
Sallan SE, Zinberg NE & Frei E (1975) Antiemetic effect of delta-9-tetrahydrocannabinol in patients receiving cancer chemotherapy. *New England Journal of Medicine* **293:** 795–797.
Samaranayake LP, Calman KC, Ferguson MM et al (1984) The oral carriage of yeasts and coliforms in patients on cytotoxic therapy. *Journal of Oral Pathology* **13:** 390–393.
Samuels ML, Selig DE, Ogden S, Grant C & Brown B (1981) IV hyperalimentation and

chemotherapy for stage III testicular cancer. A randomised study. *Cancer Treatment Reports* **65:** 615–627.
Schein PS, Macdonald JS, Waters CN & Haidak D (1974) Nutritional complications of cancer and its treatment. *Seminars in Oncology* **2:** 337–347.
Schwartz GF, Green HL, Bendon ML, Graham WP & Blackmore WS (1971) Combined parenteral hyperalimentation and chemotherapy in the treatment of solid tumours. *American Journal of Surgery* **121:** 169–173.
Shapot VS & Blinov VA (1974) Blood glucose levels and gluconeogenesis in animals bearing transplantable tumours. *Cancer Research* **34:** 1827–1832.
Souchon EA, Copeland EM, Watson P & Dudrick SJ (1975) Intravenous hyperalimentation as an adjunct to cancer chemotherapy with 5-fluorouracil. *Journal of Surgical Research* **18:** 451–454.
Sporn MB & Todero GJ (1980) Autocrine secretion and malignant transformation of cells. *New England Journal of Medicine* **303:** 878–880.
Steiger E, Oram-Smith J, Miller E, Kuo L & Vars HM (1975) Effects of nutrition on tumour growth and tolerance to chemotherapy. *Journal of Surgical Research* **18:** 455–461.
Stein TP (1978) Cachexia, gluconeogenesis and progressive weight loss in cancer patients. *Journal of Theoretical Biology* **73:** 51–59.
Stewart AG & Begg RW (1953) Systemic effects of tumours in torceren rats II. Effect on weight of carcass, adrenals, thymus, liver and spleen. *Cancer Research* **13:** 556–559.
Strain AJ (1979) Cancer cachexia in man: a review. *Investigative Cell Pathology* **2:** 181–193.
Theologides A (1977) Cancer cachexia. In Winick M (ed.) *Current concepts in nutrition* Vol. 6, pp 75–94. New York: Wiley.
Valdivesio M, Bodey GP, Benjamin RS et al (1981) Role of intravenous hyperalimentation as an adjunct to intensive chemotherapy for small cell bronchogenic carcinoma. *Cancer Treatment Reports* **65** (supplement 5): 145–150.
Valerio D, Overett L, Malcolm A & Blackburn GL (1978) Nutritional support for cancer patients receiving abdominal and pelvic radiotherapy. A randomised prospective clinical experiment of intravenous versus oral feeding. *Surgical Forum* **29:** 145–148.
Von Meyenfeldt MF, Chance WT & Fischer JE (1982) Correlation of changes in brain indoleamine metabolism with onset of anorexia in rats. *American Journal of Surgery* **143:** 133–138.
Von Meyenfeldt MF & Soeters PB (1986) Mechanisms of anorexia in cancer and potential ways for intervention. In Calman KC & Fearon KCH (eds) *Nutritional Support for the Cancer Patient*, pp 293–306. London: WB Saunders.
Walsh TD, Bowman KB & Jackson GP (1983) Dietary intake of advanced cancer patients. *Human Nutrition: Applied Nutrition* **37A:** 41–45.
Warburg O (1930) *Metabolism of tumours*. Translated by F Dickens. London: Arnold Constable.
Warren S (1932) The immediate causes of death in cancer. *American Journal of Medical Science* **184:** 610–616.
Waterhouse C (1974) Lactate metabolism in patients with cancer. *Cancer* **33:** 66–71.
Waterhouse C & Kemperman JH (1971) Carbohydrate metabolism in subjects with cancer. *Cancer Research* **31:** 1273–1278.
Waterhouse C (1974) Lactate metabolism in patients with cancer. *Cancer* **33:** 66–71.
Waterhouse C, Jeanpretre N & Keilson J (1979) Gluconeogenesis from alanine in patients with progressive malignant disease. *Cancer Research* **39:** 1968–1972.
Weinhouse S (1982) Changing perceptions of carbohydrate metabolism in tumours. In Arnott MS, Van Eys J & Wang YM (eds) *Molecular Interrelations of Nutrition and Cancer*, pp 167–181. New York: Raven Press.
Wesdorp RIC (1986) Role of abnormal metabolism in the aetiology of cancer cachexia. In Calman KC & Fearon KCH (eds) *Nutritional Support for the Cancer Patient*, pp 307–316. London: WB Saunders.
Willox JC, Corr J, Shaw J, Richardson M & Calman KC (1984) Prednisolone as an appetite stimulant in patients with cancer. *British Medical Journal* **288:** 27.
Wilmore DW (1983) Alterations in protein carbohydrate and fat metabolism in injured and septic patients. *Journal of the American College of Nutrition* **2:** 3–13.

4

The treatment of nausea and vomiting induced by cytotoxic drugs

M. SOUKOP
D. CUNNINGHAM

It is clear from most people's experience that many different pathologies cause vomiting. It is noticeable that the emetic process is associated with a common sequence of physiological activities such as yawning, excessive salivation and nausea. Co-ordinated motor activities affecting the respiratory, gastrointestinal and abdominal muscles lead to retching and actual vomiting. In view of the wide aetiologies leading to vomiting, it seems unlikely that they are governed by a common mechanism; however, three general components appear to hold true for all.

1. Afferent pathways relaying the emetic signal to the central nervous system.
2. A central reception, recognition and processing area or areas which integrates the emetic signal, which then emerges from the central nervous system (vomiting centre).
3. Efferent pathways which co-ordinate respiratory, gastrointestinal and abdominal movements accompanying emesis.

In this chapter, we shall describe some of the important features of the anatomy, physiology and pharmacology of emesis, particularly as it relates to chemotherapy-induced nausea and vomiting. We shall also review the drugs available for the treatment of cytotoxic emesis with some additional comments on psychological factors, such as anticipatory nausea and vomiting.

ANATOMY, PHYSIOLOGY AND PHARMACOLOGY

Afferent pathways

A variety of afferent pathways transmit the emetic signal from the end organ receptor.

The gastrointestinal tract

In animal experiments stimulation of the vagus nerve branches supplying the stomach has been shown to elicit vomiting. A similar response can be provoked by gastric distension, especially of the pylorus. Chemical 'irritation' of the gastric mucosa by nitrogen mustard (mustine hydrochloride) or copper sulphate in experimental models also produces the vomiting response. This can be abolished by cutting the gastric branches of the vagus, but is unaffected by dividing the splanchnic nerves. In vomiting resulting from intestinal obstruction, biliary colic and cardiac pain the stimulus appears to be transmitted via sympathetic pathways.

Chemoreceptor trigger zone

In a series of classical experiments, Borison and Wang (1953) identified an area separate from the co-ordinating vomiting centre. This area is situated in the floor of the fourth ventricle within the area postrema (AP). Histologically, it resembles the carotid body and is not part of the brain. The AP exchanges solutes directly with the cerebrospinal fluid by means of free flow through pericapillary spaces which are continuous with the subarachnoid fluid space. Equally, it is in direct contact with circulatory blood and is thus outside the blood–brain barrier.

Little is known about the function of this chemoreceptor trigger zone (CTZ). However, experimental systems show that it is sensitive to apomorphine and that ablation of the CTZ abolishes the vomiting response in dogs. The response to intragastric copper sulphate remains intact. The chemosensitive receptors in the CTZ remain uncertain and it is curious that the area can respond to so many widely divergent chemical structures. Afferent pathways to the CTZ pass through the tractus solitarius and its nucleus and efferent pathways exit via the nucleus ambiguus and the dorsal motor nuclei of the vagus. In these pathways there are receptors for a variety of neurotransmitters, including muscarinic cholinergic, histamine H_1, dopamine D-2 and opioid receptors. Over 17 probable neurotransmitters have been identified in or near the nucleus of the tractus solitarius and the AP. Hence the mechanisms involved are likely to be extremely complex and, as yet, remain undefined, apart from the overall responses to certain classes of antiemetics on some receptors.

Labyrinth

Motion sickness and vomiting associated with labyrinthitis are mediated via impulses from the labyrinth along the vestibular nerve to the lateral medulla (Reason and Brand, 1975).

Other afferents

Electrical stimulation of the hypothalamus in the cat can sometimes induce vomiting which may be delayed (Borison and Wang, 1953). Clearly, higher centres also have input to the vomiting centre.

Vomiting centre

Although the concept of a vomiting centre had long been postulated, Borison and Wang were the first to identify the importance of certain sites of the lateral reticular formation of the medulla (Borison and Wang, 1949; Borison, 1959). Stimulation of adjacent areas in their experiments resulted in some vomiting associated responses, including salivation, spasmodic respiratory movements, forced inspiration and vasomotor reactions. A series of recent electrical stimulation experiments by Miller and Wilson (1983), failed to unequivocally localize a single vomiting centre. However, the concept of a vomiting centre remains, and since its function is that of co-ordinating the multiple physiological reactions in vomiting it may be a number of adjacent, closely inter-related sites rather than a single zone.

Efferent pathways

The efferent component to vomiting is the transmission of signals from the lateral medulla via somatic efferent pathways controlling respiratory and abdominal muscles and visceral efferent components, modifying gastric tone and motility, and also autonomic efferents producing salivation, pallor and sweating.

The vagus has an important role in transmitting signals to the abdominal musculature. Although a number of neurotransmitters such as vasoactive intestinal peptide, purine nucleotides and dopamine have been suggested to be involved, a number of other candidates also exist, perhaps with different neurotransmitters or combinations of neurotransmitters being involved in the different somatic, visceral and autonomic responses.

CYTOTOXIC DRUGS AND EMESIS

Virtually all cytotoxic drugs can cause nausea and vomiting; however, the emetic potential can vary greatly from a few patients affected mildly to universal vomiting of considerable severity which may be the dose-limiting toxicity for the drug. Equally, the time lag from treatment to the onset of vomiting can be quite considerable.

Cytotoxic drugs such as the antimetabolites and vinca alkaloids, which generally interfere with DNA synthesis or mitosis, have low emetic potential. Drugs primarily inhibiting RNA and protein synthesis cause much more severe vomiting. Although the onset of symptoms tends to be quicker in the latter group, i.e. 1–6 h compared to 6–12 h, in the former this is less clear-cut. Thus cisplatin, which is almost universally emetogenic, may also induce late (12–24 h) as well as early vomiting. Perhaps two separate mechanisms are involved. Equally, the vomiting induced by some drugs is significantly later than the peak drug levels at which the CTZ would be affected. The explanation of this is unknown. The mechanism of emetine-induced vomiting is of particular interest as it inhibits brain protein synthesis. Continued brain protein synthesis is known to be involved in neurotransmitter function. Harris (1982) hypothesized that cytotoxic drugs may inhibit enkephalin-degrading enzymes in the CTZ. If these enzymes were inhibited, enkephalin levels would rise, exciting emetic receptors perhaps through some dopamine neuronal interaction. As yet, this theory has not been tested but early work by our group (Forrest et al, 1987) has found significant rises above normal in β-endorphin just prior to the onset of nausea and vomiting, with no rise in patients without symptoms. In contrast, no rise above the normal range was found in [met]enkephalin levels. In addition, the theory proposed by Harris seems unlikely as cisplatin is devoid of any significant enkephalinase-inhibiting activity in vitro. Furthermore, a potent enkephalinase inhibitor thiorphan does not induce emesis in either dogs or humans. Also, the most recent experience with 5-hydroxytryptamine M-receptor ($5\text{-}HT_3$) blockers in animals (Miner and Sanger 1986) and in man (Cunningham et al 1987a) suggest that this is the most important receptor for cytotoxic-drug-induced emesis and may be the final, common pathway of emesis.

ANTIEMETICS

The use of antiemetics in the field of chemotherapy has to date had three fairly distinct phases.

Prior to the 1960s the use of the available agents phenothiazines and antihistamines was largely empirical. The chemotherapy was in modern terms fairly ineffective and generally of low emetic potential.

In the mid- and late-1970s more effective and toxic combination chemotherapy regimes had been developed. Equally, the available antiemetic spectrum had increased to include the butyrophenone analogue domperidone, the naturally occurring cannabinoid, Δ^9-tetrahydrocannabinol (THC) and the synthetic cannabinoids nabilone and levonantradol.

The third phase was stimulated by the introduction into oncological practice of the highly emetogenic cisplatin. New strategies of antiemetic control had to be devised, hence the use of high-dose metoclopramide, steroids and combinations of antiemetics of different groups. The number of trials of antiemetic therapies reported have increased greatly as part of the search for antiemetic control. This good control is essential as emesis is perceived by patients to be the most distressing side-effect of therapy and may in some patients result in rejection of further treatment and impairment of survival.

Peroutka and Snyder (1982) pointed out that antiemetic drugs variously exhibit histamine H_1, muscarinic (cholinergic) and dopamine D-2 blocking actions, and antiemetics currently available can be classified accordingly, with the addition of the $5\text{-}HT_3$ receptor antagonists.

1. Anti-dopamine agents—phenothiazines, butyrophenones, domperidone, metoclopramide.
2. Histamine H_1 blocking agents—cyclizine, cinnarizine.
3. Muscarinic anti-cholinergic agents—hyoscine.

4. Opioid receptors—cannabinoids and related agents—THC, nabilone.
5. Cortico-steroids.
6. H_2 receptor antagonists.
7. Benzodiazepines—lorazepam.
8. 5-HT_3 receptor antagonists—GR38032F (Glaxo, Ware); ICS 205-930 (Sandoz Basel) (Leibundgut and Lancranjan, 1987); BRL24924 (Beecham Pharmaceuticals) (Andrews and Hawthorn, 1987).

DESIGN OF STUDIES

Undoubtedly, antiemetic studies are very difficult to do well. The antiemetic treatment is only one component of a very complex patient care system. In addition, the antiemetic treatment is secondary in importance to the correct treatment of the disease. It is often not possible for the needs of the antiemetic study to take precedence over other factors in deciding how the patient should be treated. The lack of a very dependable animal model, because of wide species variability and susceptibility to emetic agents, presents further difficulties in the screening for new antiemetics. Even in human studies, owing to the subjective nature of many of these unpleasant side-effects, no accepted universal standards exist. Hence the design of antiemetic studies needs to be carefully planned and rigorously carried out. Certain features are of major importance when considering such studies.

1. The study needs to be randomized and preferably double-blind. However, the side-effects of the antiemetics themselves may make it obvious to both staff and patients which antiemetic they are receiving. The numbers of patients in the study must be adequate, the study end-points clearly defined, and the techniques of analysis appropriate.
2. The emetogenic potential of the chemotherapies involved, if not identical, must be as close as possible.
3. Because of the subjective nature of many of the chemotherapy-induced effects, a cross-over design eliminates much of the individual patient variation. Ideally, an ABA versus BAB design should be used, but this is often impractical as many patients are unwilling to return to a less effective antiemetic. Studies must, however, be assessed for possibility of order preference.
4. Patients included in antiemetic studies should be new patients to avoid the possibility of anticipatory vomiting.
5. Studies of antiemetics, even those planned as out-patient regimes, should be studied in the context of the trial as in-patients, to allow the same trained observer to assess the patient and to obtain post-treatment data early to avoid errors.
6. Assessment of antiemetic response is complex and difficult but should include separate evaluation of nausea, retching and vomiting. Episodes of vomiting can be counted but can present difficulties in being accurate in some patients. Times of onset and termination of symptoms are essential. Subjective evaluations may use techniques such as linear ana-

logue scales. Patient preference between the two arms of a cross-over study and the reasons for it are very valuable. All side-effects of antiemetics must be recorded.

PHENOTHIAZINES

Phenothiazines are probably among the most widely used antiemetic agents. All the current phenothiazines have a similar base structure, differing only in two substituted positions. Side-effects and potency of the phenothiazines depend upon the various substitutions. Prochlorperazine and thiethylperazine, which have been found to have the highest antiemetic potency and least degree of sedation, have a piperazine group in the R1 side chain. Apart from sedation, the most distressing side-effect of the phenothiazines are extrapyramidal reactions; these are more common with a piperazine group side chain than with the aliphatic side chain. This acute reaction can be controlled by intravenous treatment with diphenhydramine. Phenothiazines are thought to act by blocking dopamine receptors, predominantly in the chemoreceptor trigger zone. Thus their ability to act against the emesis of agents causing vomiting through pathways other than the dopamine receptor may be limited.

Prochlorperazine has been evaluated extensively, a recent review listing 27 comparative studies involving 1567 patients (Bakowski, 1984). The findings from these are generally consistent in showing prochlorperazine to be superior to a placebo, other phenothiazines and benzquinamide. Only one study found no difference between prochlorperazine and placebo. Most of the earlier studies involved patients receiving chemotherapy regimens of relatively low emetic potential and prochlorperazine is of limited clinical value for regimens of intermediate or high emetogenicity. Chlorpromazine is an effective antiemetic against chemotherapy regimens that do not contain cisplatin (Cunningham et al, 1985a). In our experience 25 mg i.m. every 4 h beginning at the same time as chemotherapy and continued for 12 h completely controlled nausea and vomiting in over 40% of patients. However, its use is associated with sedation in 70% of patients and therefore it cannot easily be given in the out-patient clinic. Chlorpromazine is not useful against cisplatin induced emesis (Cunningham et al, 1985a).

BUTYROPHENONES

Haloperidol and droperidol are the best known of the original members of this group, the latter being synthesized in 1961. These compounds are potent neuroleptics and, like the phenothiazines, probably exert their antiemetic properties through dopamine antagonism and the inhibition of dopamine receptors in the CTZ. They are generally considered to be more active in this regard than the phenothiazines while producing less sedation. The butyrophenones also may cause akathisias or restlessness (restless legs syndrome), and more rarely extrapyramidal reactions. Effects upon the cardiovascular and respiratory systems are minimal. The drugs are extensively metabolized by the liver by hepatic oxidation and N alkylation with a high hepatic extraction ratio. The high clearance of the drug results in a short $t_{1/2}$, hence the drugs may need to be administered frequently or preferably by infusion. However, despite the pharmacokinetic data, droperidol has a more prolonged duration of pharmacologic action than would be predicted. This may imply a slow dissociation of droperidol from its receptor, or its retention in the brain. Ten publications (Bakowski, 1984) give details of trials in which droperidol, as a single agent, has been compared to other antiemetics in the management of cytotoxin-induced emesis. These studies involve 178 patients during 259 courses of chemotherapy.

Nine of the studies involved cisplatin-containing schedules. In three of these, other antiemetics were superior to droperidol. In the remainder, droperidol was superior or equal in effect to the reference antiemetic. Rather surprisingly, studies in which higher doses, i.e. 4 mg/m^2, four-hourly, of droperidol were used, showed droperidol was inferior to the reference antiemetics. However, droperidol overall is less than optimum in cisplatin-induced nausea and vomiting. Only four extrapyramidal reactions were noted in these studies. Droperidol is generally given as an intravenous infusion of 1–1.5 mg/h over 8 h with chemotherapy or can be given as two separate i.v. infusions (the first of which is given with chemotherapy) of 0.5–1 mg/m^2 with a time interval between infusions of 30 min.

DOMPERIDONE

Domperidone, a benzimidazole derivative, is chemically related to the butyrophenones. Compared to metoclopramide, it has been suggested it crosses the blood–brain barrier poorly and therefore gives a lower incidence of central nervous system toxicity, including sedation and extrapyramidal reactions. The proposed mechanism of antiemetic action is the stimulation of gastric motility and blocking of peripheral dopamine receptors. Available data indicate that domperidone is superior to placebo but probably not as potent as THC or metoclopramide. It probably has only limited effects in cisplatin-containing regimens (Hamers, 1978; Huys, 1978; Swann et al, 1979; D'Souza et al, 1980; O'Meara and Mott, 1981).

A number of case reports of sudden death, cardiac arrest, or clinically significant arrhythmias in patients receiving intravenous domperidone have led to the withdrawal of the intravenous preparation of the drug. In a recent randomized trial in patients receiving chemotherapy without cisplatin, oral domperidone 20 mg three times a day was compared to oral/intravenous metoclopramide, 20 mg three times a day or oral/intravenous dexamethasone 4 mg three times a day. Domperidone emerged as intermediate between the other two in terms of antiemetic efficacy (Cunningham et al, 1987b). However, it was only able to provide complete control of nausea and vomiting in 40% of cases and therefore, given on its own, is unlikely to be sufficient. However, since it has few side-effects, it can be combined with other antiemetics, particularly dexamethasone.

METOCLOPRAMIDE

Metoclopramide is a substituted benzamide closely related to procainamide. It is thought to exert its antiemetic effect in two ways. It is a dopamine antagonist and may inhibit input to the vomiting centre from the CTZ. Metoclopramide is effective in dogs given apomorphine, which induces emesis by stimulation of dopamine receptors in the CTZ. Metoclopramide also increases lower oesophageal sphincter tone, promotes gastric emptying and accelerates small bowel transit, thus reducing gastric stasis and reflux. Metoclopramide has the ability to reduce vomiting due to the intragastric administration of copper sulphate.

Low dose or conventional dose metoclopramide was less effective when compared to prochlorperazine in humans and was, in some studies, little better than or equal to placebo. Gralla et al (1981) renewed interest in the drug by the safe use of high doses with a much improved antiemetic profile.

In doses of 2–3 mg/kg two-hourly commencing 30 min before chemotherapy and continuing to a total of 10 mg/kg, they demonstrated in two studies, in patients receiving 120 mg/m^2 of cisplatin, superiority of metoclopramide against placebo and prochlorperazine, the mean number of episodes of emesis being 1.0 vs 10.5 and 1.5 vs 12.0, respectively. This improvement was achieved in this study at the cost of mild sedation and only one extrapyramidal reaction. This result has been confirmed in a number of other studies with relatively small numbers of patients.

Cunningham et al (1985a) demonstrated in a randomized study of high-dose metoclopramide against chlorpromazine the superiority of antiemetic control by metoclopramide only in patients receiving cisplatin. The observer-assessed superiority was supported by the patient preference for metoclopramide.

Gralla et al (1984) compared metoclopramide 10 mg/kg in divided doses to THC 50 mg/m^2 in divided doses, in patients receiving cisplatin 120 mg/m^2. Metoclopramide was superior with respect to median vomiting episodes (1 versus 8) and exerted a major antiemetic effect in 86% compared to 21% for THC.

The Edinburgh group (Warrington et al, 1986) among others, have suggested that high dose metoclopramide was less effective than initially reported. In consequence, they investigated pharmacokinetically in a randomized study intermittent versus loading dose with continuous infusion of high dose metoclopramide in order to optimize the antiemetic potential of the drug. The loading dose followed by continuous infusion was clearly superior in providing a steady and adequate plasma concentration over an eight-hour period. This also resulted in improved antiemetic control.

Meyer et al (1984) have also studied plasma concentration of metoclopramide in relation to antiemetic control in patients receiving cisplatin. Patients in whom the plasma concentration was equal to or greater than 850 ng/ml 6 h post-chemotherapy, achieved 78% excellent, 18% partial antiemetic control, compared to 0% excellent and 42% partial control with less than 850 ng/ml plasma concentration. In patients receiving chemotherapy other than cisplatin such levels might not be necessary, as Strum et al (1984) found that 20 mg i.v. repeated two-hourly for six doses was as effective as higher doses. However, a recent study of intermediate dose metoclopramide (20 mg three times a day orally) showed it to be an ineffective antiemetic (Cunningham et al, 1987b).

The most common side-effect of high dose metoclopramide is mild to moderate sedation, also diarrhoea has been quite frequently reported. However, less common but of greater severity, are the central nervous system toxicities. These relate to the extrapyramidal system and may be severe dystonia or mild akathisia (restlessness). The paper by Kris et al (1983) examines the incidence of extrapyramidal reactions in 452 patients receiving high dose metoclopramide. The most striking feature was the well-recognized sensitivity of the younger patient, with six incidents in 22 patients (27.3%) in the age range 15–29 years, compared to eight incidents in 430 patients (1.8%) in the age range 30–72 years.

All workers have confirmed the effectiveness of diphenhydramine 50 mg i.v. to completely abolish the side-effect within 5 min. In the young patient given high dose metoclopramide as an antiemetic, prophylactic diphenhydramine has been suggested.

Occasional cases have been reported of tardive dyskinesia associated with short-term high dose metoclopramide (Breitbart, 1986).

CANNABINOIDS

Following anecdotal reports of the value of marijuana in alleviating chemotherapy-induced nausea and vomiting, a clinical research programme isolated THC, the most active of more than 50 cannabinoids in the plant *Cannabis sativa* L. THC taken orally is variably but poorly absorbed of the order of 5–10%. It is bound tightly to plasma proteins. The drug is extensively metabolized in the liver to numerous 11-hydroxylated metabolites, a few of which are still psychoactive.

Cannabinoids have many physiological actions (Ashton, 1987), including psychotropic effects, hypnotic, tranquillizing, antiemetic, anticonvulsant and analgesic. They also lower intra-ocular pressure, increase appetite and affect the cardiovascular system, causing tachycardia or hypotension, respiratory, reproductive and immune symptoms. Acute exposure can precipitate anxiety, panic, depersonalization and schizophreniform, manic and confusional psychoses. Certain personality characteristics may predispose to such acute reactions and care must be taken in patient selection.

The high lipid-solubility of THC contributes to its relatively long plasma half-life as the fat stores in the body act as a slow drug-release mechanism. Nabilone, a synthetic cannabinoid, was selected after screening over 700 analogues. Levonantradol, another synthetic cannabinoid, was withdrawn after initial trials. Cannabinoids are thought to inhibit efferent pathways from the vomiting centre and may, in addition, inhibit prostaglandins in synthesis. A number of studies have indicated that the antiemetic efficacy of these agents often coincides with some degree of central nervous system toxicity, recognized as dysphoria, sedation and confusion. The effectiveness of THC and nabilone have been demonstrated in a number of controlled studies and THC has been shown to be superior to prochlorperazine and placebo.

Sallan et al (1980) investigated the effectiveness of THC versus prochlorperazine in the double-blind randomized study. The THC dosage was 10 mg/m^2 orally, 1 h before and 3 and 7 h post-chemotherapy. Prochlorperazine was given at a dose of 10 mg orally, using the same time schedule. The study consisted of 84 patients receiving cytotoxic chemotherapy. Complete control of nausea and vomiting was achieved in 36 of 70 patients on THC (46%), compared to 16 of 78 (21%) of those on prochlorperazine. A relationship between the complete control of nausea and vomiting and attainment of a 'high' were shown. Out of 41 patients in whom a 'high' occurred, 32 had complete control of nausea and vomiting, compared to only four of 38 with no 'high'. A similar correlation of antiemetic effect and mood alteration has been noted in other studies (Orr et al, 1980; Lucas and Laszlo, 1980).

Some of the variability of the effect of oral THC may be attributed to the variability in absorption and hence failure to achieve therapeutic levels. Sallan et al (1980) noted a relationship between age and complete response, with total control of nausea and vomiting in 15 out of 20 courses in patients 20 years or less, compared to 21 of 59 courses in patients 21 years or older. This difference was significant, $P=0.004$. The mean age of Sallan's whole group was 32.5 years and only four out of 24 patients were described as having significant drug toxicity. Additionally, Sallan's group suggested that THC was generally effective regardless of emetogenic challenge, although other workers have found much less benefit with more intensive chemotherapies. Frytak et al (1979), in a group of 116 patients with a median age of 61 years, using a dose of THC of 15 mg orally, 2 h before, and 2 and 8 h after chemotherapy, on day 1, and 30 min before meals on days 2, 3 and 4 of a 4-day chemotherapy schedule. Although THC was demonstrated to be reasonably effective in terms of controlling nausea and vomiting, excessive sedation and co-ordination problems, as well as dysphoria, were frequently noted and 32% refused to continue because of these side-effects. It has been suggested that increased toxicity from THC increases with age. However, if an absolute relationship existed between toxicity and benefit, THC should also be more effective in the older patients.

This is not our experience and probably relates more to a lower tolerance of dysphoria in older patients. In a study of 55 patients by Orr et al (1980), THC, 7 mg/m^2 orally 1 h before and 4, 8, 12 and 16 h post-chemotherapy, was found to be more effective than prochlorperazine at the same dose and schedule in the group receiving Adriamycin (doxorubicin), 5-fluorouracil and cyclophosphamide. In patients receiving BCNU (carmustine) or nitrogen mustard, adequate antiemetic control was not achieved in either group. This lack of effectiveness by THC in more intensive schedules was also suggested by Lucas and Laszlo (1980) in patients receiving variable doses of cisplatin.

Nabilone is formed by a substitution of a ketone for a methyl group in the 9 position of the C ring and also changes in the structure of the side chain. It is not metabolized to THC. Nabilone is felt to have less cardiovascular and central nervous system side-effects.

Nabilone was introduced into clinical trial in 1976. Early studies indicated reduced nausea and vomiting and also patient preference against placebo, low-dose metoclopramide and prochlorperazine. A randomized study of oral nabilone, 1 mg twice a day, with oral prochlorperazine, 5 mg twice a day, versus nabilone alone (Cunningham et al, 1985b) showed, as expected, no significant differences in nausea, vomiting, appetite or adverse side-effects of the antiemetics, apart from those of the central nervous system. The incidence of dysphoria/hallucinations in the combined arm was only 3% compared to 39% using single agent nabilone. The patients in this study were receiving non-platinum-containing regimens, the antiemetic complete control being good at 85% and 74%, respectively.

However, in an extension of this work, we were unable to show nabilone and prochlorperazine to be better than high dose metoclopramide and dexamethasone in patients receiving cisplatin combinations. The complete control of vomiting with nabilone and Stemetil (prochlorperazine mesylate) was 31.5% compared to 55.6% with high dose metoclopramide and dexamethasone (Cunningham et al, 1987c). Nevertheless, for those patients receiving the cisplatin analogue carboplatin, nabilone and prochlorperazine was the preferred antiemetic.

STEROIDS

Dexamethasone and methylprednisolone as a single agent has antiemetic activity (Lee, 1981; Kolaric and Roth, 1983). In a recent study, oral dexamethasone 4 mg three times a day (with one intravenous dose of 4 mg with chemotherapy) given for 3 days and then tailed off over the next 2 days, was able to control nausea and vomiting in 75% of patients given chemotherapy regimens without cisplatin. It was also effective in patients who had failed to respond to domperidone (Cunningham et al, 1987b). The mechanism of action of dexamethasone is unknown but clearly deserves further investigation.

In patients receiving cisplatin, the combination of dexamethasone and high dose metoclopramide improved control of vomiting and retching and enhanced the recovery from nausea (Allan et al, 1984). This study and others have shown a reduction in the incidence of diarrhoea when the combination is used.

An interesting study by Strum et al (1985) noted that metoclopramide plus dexamethasone, although statistically not different to metoclopramide alone in controlling emesis, was significantly preferred by patients in a ratio of 6:1.

LORAZEPAM

Lorazepam is a member of the benzodiazepine family of anxiolytic agents. Its potential value in the treatment of emesis induced by cytotoxic drugs was first recognized when it was given at a dose of 4–5 mg i.v. immediately before chemotherapy in combination with perphenazine 5 mg i.v. which was given 1 h before chemotherapy to a group of seven patients with emesis refractory to standard antiemetic therapy (Maher, 1981). Vomiting was markedly reduced in six of the seven patients and in three out of four patients anticipatory vomiting was prevented. However all patients experienced significant drowsiness but in general were easily rousable 5–15 min after lorazepam. In a subsequent study, lorazepam 2.5 mg/m^2 given by slow i.v. injection 30 min before chemotherapy was compared to high dose metoclopramide in 19 patients receiving combination chemotherapy by regimens that included cisplatin (Bowcock et al, 1984). Antiemetic control was similar with both antiemetics but patients preferred lorazepam because of its anxiolytic effect. All patients given lorazepam experienced moderate or marked sedation. Lorazepam has also been given sublingually at a dose of 0.05 mg/kg to the nearest 1 mg 30 min before chemotherapy and appears to be an effective antiemetic (Bishop et al, 1984).

Lorazepam is undoubtedly a useful antiemetic. Its major drawback is sedation which essentially precludes its use in an out-patient setting. However, for patients with anticipatory vomiting it can be particularly useful. It should also be possible to combine lorazepam at a dose of 1 mg/m^2 given 30 min before chemotherapy with oral dexamethasone 4 mg four times a day for 3 days as a means of reducing sedative side effects while maintaining the antiemetic effect.

5-HYDROXYTRYPTAMINE M-RECEPTOR (5-HT$_3$) ANTAGONISTS

Although drugs such as nabilone, dexamethasone and high dose metoclopramide have made a significant contribution to improving the control of emesis induced by cytotoxic drugs, none is totally effective or devoid of side-effects. The pathophysiology of nausea and vomiting related to cytotoxic drugs is not fully understood. Many of the agents used to treat emesis are dopamine antagonists because the model classically used to test antiemetics was apomorphine-induced emesis in the dog. This model utilizes the dopaminergic pathways. Metoclopramide, the substituted benzamide, is a potent dopamine antagonist, but at a conventional dose (Cunningham et al 1987b) it is not very effective against chemotherapy-induced emesis. Escalating the dose of metoclopramide improves antiemetic control (Cunningham et al 1985a) but leads to extrapyramidal reactions in up to 15% of patients (Cunningham et al 1987c). At these higher, more therapeutically useful, doses it antagonizes 5-HT at the 5-HT$_3$ receptor (Fozard, 1984; Schultz-Delerieu, 1979; Miner and Sanger, 1986). Miner and Sanger (1986) therefore suggested that this might be the mechanism by which metoclopramide is antiemetic. 5-HT$_3$ receptors have so far only been located in the periphery, notably on vagal afferents and enteric neurones (Fozard, 1984; Richardson et al 1986).

In animals, selective 5-HT$_3$ antagonists (Fozard, 1984; Miner and Sanger, 1986) have been shown to control vomiting induced by several different cytotoxic drugs. GR38032F (Glaxo Group Research Ltd., Ware) is a selective 5-HT_3 antagonist (Figure 1) which has been shown to be an effective antiemetic against cisplatin-induced emesis in the ferret (Costall et al, 1987). The ferret model of emesis is now regarded as one of the best models available for the testing of antiemetics against cytotoxic drugs and is certainly of more clinical relevance than the model which utilizes apomorphine-induced vomiting in the dog.

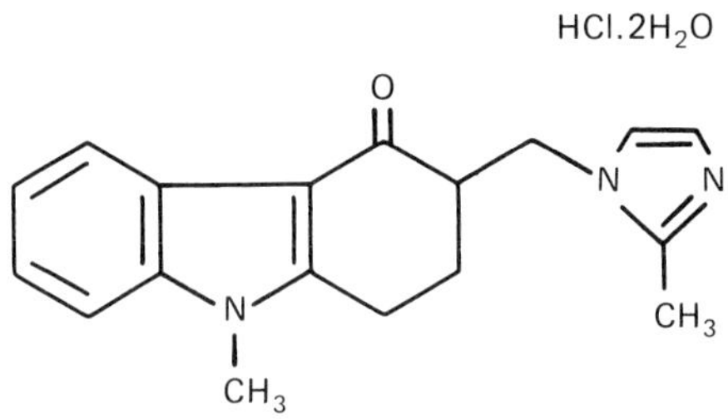

Figure 1. Structure of GR38032F. 1,2,3,9-Tetrahydro-3-((2-methylimidazol-1-yl)methyl)-9-methyl-4H-carbazol-4-one HCl dihydrate.

In healthy volunteers, GR38032F was shown to be well tolerated as a single intravenous dose up to 128 μg/kg and a single oral dose up to 160 μg/kg and 75 patients received repeat oral dosing up to 8 mg twice daily for one month with negligible toxicity. The half-life of GR38032F was established in normal subjects as 3–6 h and the bioavailability of the oral compound was good at 71% (Glaxo Group Research, unpublished data). On the basis of these data and the animal studies, a schedule of administration for the treatment of emesis caused by cytotoxic drugs was devised as follows: 4 mg to be given intravenously with chemotherapy and at the same time 4 mg to be given orally. The oral dose to be repeated 5 h and 10 h later.

Using this schedule, 15 patients with nausea and vomiting induced by a variety of cytotoxic drugs (excluding cisplatin) which had proven refractory to standard antiemetic therapy (dexamethasone alone or in combination with domperidone or metoclopramide) were treated. In 31 courses of chemotherapy, only one patient experienced vomiting. The only side-effects possibly related to antiemetic treatment were dryness of the mouth in one patient and mild sedation in another (Cunningham et al, 1987a). This is in sharp contrast to previous experience in the control of refractory vomiting using a multiple antiemetic combination which, although successful, resulted in an escalation of side-effects, particularly drowsiness (Plezia et al, 1984).

The only other 5-HT_3 receptor antagonist which has been reported to be antiemetic against cytotoxic drugs in humans is ICS 205-930 (Sandoz Ltd. Basel) but side-effects were more frequent (headache in nine of 47 courses, mild sedation in seven of 47 courses) than with GR38032F (Leibundgut and Lancranjan, 1987). Other 5-HT_3 antagonists are currently being investigated in humans and the results are awaited with interest.

The mechanism of action of these 5-HT_3 receptor blockers has not yet been fully established. Although blockade of peripheral receptors may be important, evidence from nerve section techniques indicate that, on its own, peripheral blockade is unlikely to prevent emesis (Andrews and Hawthorn, 1987). So far, 5-HT_3 receptors have not been demonstrated in the brain but few would doubt they are there.

The 5-HT_3 receptor antagonists are a new class of antiemetic agents which are likely to make a significant contribution to the management of emesis induced by cytotoxic drugs. They may also help our understanding of the complex mechanism of the induction of nausea and vomiting related to chemotherapy.

RECOMMENDATIONS FOR CLINICAL PRACTICE

Tables 1 and 2 give guidelines for a practical approach to the problem of nausea and vomiting induced by cytotoxic drugs. They do not include any of the 5HT_3 receptor antagonists because at the time of writing these compounds are not available for routine use. In general, it is useful to divide chemotherapy regimens into those with or without cisplatin, because cisplatin combinations are universally emetogenic and are virtually always given on an in-patient basis to facilitate hyperhydration. However, the emetogenic potential of regimens without cisplatin should not be underestimated. In a group of 60 patients receiving a variety of cytotoxic regimens which did not include cisplatin, once triggered, the median duration of nausea was 3.5 days with a range of 1–14 days (Cunningham et al, 1987b). It therefore seems sensible to continue antiemetic therapy for more than 24 h, and the majority of investigators would recommend 3–5 days of treatment.

Table 1. Antiemetic schedules for patients receiving cisplatin.

Drug	Dose and schedule	Comments
Metoclopramide	2 mg/kg i.v. loading dose over the 15 min prior to chemotherapy	Diphenhydramine 30 mg i.v. may be given 30 min prior to chemotherapy to prevent extrapyramidal reactions especially in the young but will cause drowsiness
combined with	3 mg/kg i.v. infusion over the following 8 h	
Dexamethasone	20 mg i.v. with chemotherapy	Give over 4–5 min otherwise patients experience burning and paraesthesia in the perineum
Lorazepam	2.5 mg/m^2 i.v. over 30 min before chemotherapy	
combined with Dexamethasone	20 mg i.v. with chemotherapy and 4 mg four times a day for 3 days after chemotherapy	

Table 2. Antiemetic schedules for patients receiving chemotherapy regimens without cisplatin.

Drug	Dose and schedule	Comments
Dexamethasone	8 mg i.v. with chemotherapy. At the same time give an oral dose of 4 mg to be repeated 6-hourly for 48 h and then reduced to 2 mg four times a day orally for 48 h and 1 mg four times a day orally for 24 h, then stop.	
Dexamethasone as above combined with Domperidine	20 mg four times a day orally for 5 days	
Dexamethasone as above combined with Lorazepam	1 mg/m² i.v. over 15 min before chemotherapy	Particularly useful with anticipatory vomiting
Nabilone, Prochlorperazine	Nabilone 1 mg twice daily orally. Prochlorperazine 5 mg twice daily orally to a maximum of 4 dosages	Giving both drugs together has in our experience reduced the incidence of dysphoria. Predosing 6–12 h prior to therapy
Dexamethasone	8 mg–20 mg i.v.	Given 30 min prior to therapy

For patients with emesis refractory to first line antiemetic therapy, antiemetic combinations should be tried and domperidine suppositories 30 mg three times a day are occasionally of value. Chlorpromazine 25 mg i.m. repeated every 4 h as necessary is also occasionally useful.

ANTICIPATORY NAUSEA AND VOMITING

Repeated cycles of chemotherapy that are accompanied by nausea and vomiting may result in the problem of anticipatory nausea and vomiting. This can be defined as nausea or vomiting prior to or in anticipation of chemotherapy administration.

Estimates of the numbers of patients affected vary widely from 9 to 65%. This variability will depend on a number of factors including, most importantly, the intensity of the chemotherapy schedule. It has been reported that in patients with severe post-treatment nausea and vomiting over 70% experienced anticipatory vomiting (Wilcox et al, 1982). These effects may cause some patients to decline further treatment.

Morrow (1982) identified, using multivariate analysis, a number of factors which seemed especially important in the development of anticipatory nausea and vomiting:

(a) the severity of post-chemotherapy vomiting;
(b) the duration of nausea;
(c) the number of courses associatory with nausea and vomiting.

Trigger factors for anticipatory nausea and vomiting may include smells, tastes, sights and even thoughts of chemotherapy. I know of an incident when a patient no longer receiving chemotherapy greeted a nurse from the oncology clinic in a well-known Glasgow store with ‘How nice to see you again after all this time’, and promptly vomited at her feet. The phenomenon hence is similar to the classical Pavlovian conditioning.

Morrow also correlated previous susceptibility to motion sickness with increased rates of anticipatory nausea and vomiting (Morrow, 1985). Other predisposing factors include younger age, female—especially those receiving adjuvant chemotherapy for breast cancer (Morrow, 1984).

A study by Nerenz et al (1986) examined potential predictive factors for anticipatory nausea and vomiting in 192 patients commencing chemotherapy. Similar to the work of Morrow, post-treatment side-effects of nausea and especially vomiting, were important. They also indicated that the ability of the patient to taste the drug at the time of administration correlated positively (Nerenz et al, 1986). This view was not shared by investigators at the John Hopkins Cancer Center (Fetting et al, 1985). Nerenz et al (1986) also noted a positive correlation with high anxiety levels prior to chemotherapy. A number of recommendations can be made to help reduce the likelihood of anticipatory nausea and vomiting developing.

1. Advise patients to avoid new or strong-tasting foods during days of treatment. This should help to reduce taste aversion.
2. Advise patients to eat little prior to treatment.
3. Avoid strong-smelling cleaning fluids or air fresheners in treatment areas.
4. Follow-up clinics should be in a different site to the treatment area.
5. Staff involved in giving chemotherapy should avoid wearing strong perfumes.
6. Most importantly, there should be good antiemetic control with initial therapy.
7. There should be early recognition of a developing problem, perhaps with the use of relaxation techniques and behaviour modification where appropriate.
8. Short-term memory loss, together with sedation, resulting from the use of lorazepam may help to ‘desensitize’ some patients to recently-developed anticipatory symptoms. The marked sedation may be unacceptable to some patients, while being welcomed by others.

A number of controlled studies have examined the role of relaxation techniques, particularly in anticipatory symptoms.

Lyles et al (1982) randomized 50 patients receiving chemotherapy to three groups:

(a) progressive muscle relaxation training and guided relaxation imagery;
(b) positive support and encouragement;
(c) no treatment control.

Those patients receiving relaxation training reported less anxiety, nausea and were less physiologically stressed. Additionally, the duration of any side-effects was reduced.

A further study (Morrow and Morrell, 1982) of 60 ambulatory cancer patients with anticipatory nausea and vomiting before their third or fourth course of chemotherapy, were randomized to:

(a) 'systematic desensitization';
(b) counselling; and
(c) no treatment arms.

Significantly more patients in group (a) had no anticipatory nausea or vomiting before courses five and six than those in group (b) $P<0.05$ or in group (c) $P<0.01$. The severity of symptoms in the remainder was also less in group (a) and the periods of nausea were also of shorter duration. No complications of the technique were noted but the 2 h of professional time for each patient in group (a) would make it a difficult technique.

OTHER TECHNIQUES

A double-blind sequential trial by Saller et al (1986) reported the enhancement of the antiemetic action of metoclopramide infusion 3.5 mg/kg against cisplatin-induced emesis by transdermal electrical nerve stimulation (TENS). TENS reduced the number of emetic episodes in 10 out of 11 subjects. Rather surprisingly, a reduction in the extrapyramidal toxicity of metoclopramide was also seen. The effect could be blocked by naloxone. These data imply the involvement of endogenous neuropeptides, serotonergic mechanisms, or both, in the action of TENS.

SUMMARY

In this chapter, the pathophysiology of nausea and vomiting induced by cytotoxic drugs is discussed. At present, the precise mechanisms remain unclear but 5-HT_3 receptors are increasingly being recognized as having a fundamental role.

The standard antiemetic combination for patients receiving chemotherapy with cisplatin is the combination of high-dose metoclopramide and dexamethasone. For other chemotherapy regimens the emphasis should be on antiemetic therapy which can be delivered in an out-patient setting. Effective antiemetics for this purpose include the combination of nabilone and prochlorperazine, oral dexamethasone and oral domperidone. The new 5-HT_3 antagonists such as GR38032F are the most exciting prospect on the horizon and preliminary clinical trials are extremely encouraging.

REFERENCES

Allan SG, Cornbleet MA, Warrington P, Leonard RCF & Smyth JF (1984) Trial of dexamethasone and high-dose metoclopramide versus placebo and high-dose metoclopramide in cisplatin-induced emesis. *Proceedings of the American Society of Clinical Oncology* **3:** 89.

Andrews PLR & Hawthorn J (1987) Evidence for an extra-abdominal site of action for the 5-HT_3 receptor antagonist BRL24924 in the inhibition of radiation-evoked emesis in the ferret. *Neuropharmacology* **26:** 1367–1370.

Ashton CH (1987) Cannabis: dangers and possible use. *British Medical Journal* **294:** 141–142.

Bakowski MT (1984) Advances in anti-emetic therapy. *Cancer Treatment Reviews* **11:** 237–256.

Bishop JF, Olver IN, Wolf MM et al (1984) Lorazepam: a randomized, double-blind, crossover study of a new antiemetic in patients receiving cytotoxic chemotherapy and prochlorperazine. *Journal of Clinical Oncology* **2:** 691–695.

Borison HL (1959) Effect of ablation of medullary emetic chemoreceptor trigger zone on vomiting responses to cerebral intraventricular injection of adrenalin, apomorphine and pilocarpine in the cat. *Journal of Physiology* **147:** 172–177.

Borison HL & Wang SC (1949) Functional localization of central co-ordinating mechanism for emesis in the cat. *Journal of Neurophysiology* **12:** 305–313.

Borison HL & Wang SC (1953) Physiology and pharmacology of vomiting. *Pharmacology Review* **5:** 193–230.

Bowcock SJ, Stockdale AD, Bolton JAR, Kang AA & Retsas S (1984) Antiemetic prophylaxis with high dose metoclopramide or lorazepam and vomiting induced by chemotherapy. *British Medical Journal* **288:** 1879.

Breitbart W (1986) Tardive dyskinesia associated with high-dose intravenous metoclopramide. *New England Journal of Medicine* **315:** 518.

Costall B, Domeney A, Gunningh SJ, Naylor RJ, Tattershall F & Tyers MB (1987) GR38032F: a potent and novel inhibitor of cisplatin-induced emesis in the ferret. *British Journal of Pharmacology* **90:** 90P.

Cunningham D, Soukop M, Gilchrist NL et al (1985a) Randomised trial of intravenous high-dose metoclopramide and intramuscular chlorpromazine in controlling nausea and vomiting induced by cytotoxic drugs. *British Medical Journal* **290:** 604–605.

Cunningham D, Forrest GJ, Soukop M, Gilchrist NL, Calder I & McArdle CS (1985b) Nabilone and prochlorperazine: a new effective combination for the treatment of emesis induced by cytotoxic drugs. *British Medical Journal* **291:** 964–965.

Cunningham D, Hawthorn J, Pople A et al (1987a) Prevention of emesis in patients receiving cytotoxic drugs by GR38032F a selective 5-HT_3 receptor antagonist. *Lancet* **i:** 1461–1463.

Cunningham D, Evans C, Gazet JC et al (1987b) Comparison of the antiemetic efficacy of domperidone metoclopramide and dexamethasone in patients receiving out-patient chemotherapy regimens. *British Medical Journal* **295:** 250.

Cunningham D, Bradley CJ, Forrest GJ et al (1987c) A randomised trial of oral nabilone and prochlorperazine compared to intravenous metoclopramide and dexamethasone in the treatment of nausea and vomiting induced by chemotherapy regimens containing cisplatin or cisplatin analogues. *European Journal of Cancer and Clinical Oncology* (in press).

D'Souza DP, Reyntjens A & Thornes RD (1980) Domperidone in the prevention of nausea and vomiting induced by anti-neoplastic agents: a threefold evaluation. *Current Therapeutic Research* **27:** 384–390.

Fetting JH, Wilcox PM, Sheidler VR, Enterline JP, Donehower RC & Grochow LB (1985) Tastes associated with parenteral chemotherapy for breast cancer. *Cancer Treatment Report* **69:** 1249–1251.

Forrest GJ, Wallace D, Cunningham D et al (1987) β-endorphine—a modulator of emesis in patients receiving chemotherapy. *British Journal of Cancer* (in press).

Fozard JR (1984) Neuronal 5-HT receptors in the periphery. *Neuropharmacology* **23:** 1473–1486.

Frytak S, Moertel CG, O'Fallon JR et al (1979) Delta-9-tetrahydrocannabinol as an antiemetic for patients receiving cancer chemotherapy. *Annals of Internal Medicine* **91:** 825–830.

Gralla RJ, Itri LM, Pisko SE et al (1981) Antiemetic efficacy of high-dose metoclopramide: randomized trials with placebo and prochlorperazine in patients with chemotherapy-induced nausea and vomiting. *New England Journal of Medicine* **305:** 905–909.

Gralla RJ, Tyson LB, Bordin LA et al (1984) Antiemetic therapy: a review of recent studies and a report of a random assignment trial comparing metoclopramide and delta-9-tetrahydrocannabinol. *Cancer Treatment Report* **68:** 163–172.

Hamers J (1978) Cytostatic therapy induced vomiting inhibited by domperidone. A double-blind cross-over study. *Biomedicine* **29:** 242–244.

Harris AL (1982) Cytotoxic-therapy-induced vomiting is mediated via enkephalin pathways. *Lancet* **i:** 714–716.

Huys J (1978) Cytostatic associated vomiting effectively inhibited by domperidone (R33818). *Cancer Chemotherapy and Pharmacology* **1:** 215–218.

Kolaric K & Roth A (1983) Methylprednisolone as an antiemetic in patients on cisplatinum chemotherapy. Results of a controlled randomized study. *Tumori* **69:** 43–46.

Kris MG, Tyson LB, Gralla RJ, Clark RA, Allan JC & Reilly LK (1983) Extra-pyramidal reactions with high-dose metoclopramide. *New England Journal of Medicine* **309:** 433–434.

Lee BJ (1981) Methylprednisolone as an antiemetic. *New England Journal of Medicine* **304:** 486.

Leibundgut U & Lancranjan I (1987) First results with ICS 205-930 (5-HT_3 receptor antagonist) in prevention of chemotherapy-induced emesis (letter). *Lancet* **i:** 1198.

Lucas VS & Laszlo J (1980) Delta-9-tetrahydrocannabinol in refractory vomiting induced by cancer chemotherapy. *Journal of American Medical Association* **243:** 1241–1243.

Lyles JN, Burish TG, Krozely MG & Oldham RK (1982) Efficacy of relaxation training and guided imagery in reducing the aversiveness of cancer chemotherapy. *Journal of Consultant Clinical Psychology* **50:** 509–524.

Maher J (1981) Intravenous lorazepam to prevent nausea and vomiting associated with cancer chemotherapy. *Lancet* **i:** 91–92.

Meyer BR, Lewis M, Drayer DE, Pasmentier M, Lonski L & Reidenberg MM (1984) Optimizing metoclopramide control of cisplatin-induced emesis. *Annals of Internal Medicine* **100:** 393–395.

Miller AD & Wilson VJ (1983) Vomiting centre reanalyzed: an electrical stimulation study. *Brain Research* **270:** 154–158.

Miner WD & Sanger GH (1986) Inhibition of cisplatin-induced vomiting by selective 5-Hydroxytryptamine M-receptor antagonism. *British Journal of Pharmacology* **88:** 497–499.

Morrow GR (1982) Prevalence and correlates of anticipatory nausea and vomiting in chemotherapy patients. *Journal of National Cancer Institute* **68:** 585–588.

Morrow GR (1984) Clinical characteristics associated with the development of anticipatory nausea and vomiting in cancer patients undergoing chemotherapy treatment. *Journal of Clinical Oncology* **2:** 1170–1176.

Morrow GR (1985) The effect of a susceptibility to motion sickness on the side-effects of cancer chemotherapy. *Cancer* **55:** 2766–2770.

Morrow GR & Morrell C (1982) Behavioural treatment for the anticipatory nausea and vomiting induced by cancer chemotherapy. *New England Journal of Medicine* **307:** 1476–1480.

Nerenz DR, Leventhal H, Easterling DV & Love RR (1986) Anxiety and drug taste as predictors of anticipatory nausea in cancer chemotherapy. *Journal of Clinical Oncology* **4:** 224–233.

O'Meara A & Mott G (1981) Domperidone as an antiemetic in paediatric oncology. *Cancer Chemotherapy and Pharmacology* **6:** 147–149.

Orr LE, McKernan JF & Bloome B (1980) Antiemetic effect of tetrahydrocannabinol compared with placebo and prochlorperazine in chemotherapy-associated nausea and emesis. *Archives of Internal Medicine* **140:** 1431–1433.

Peroutka SJ & Snyder SH (1982) Antiemetics: neurotransmitter receptor binding predicts therapeutic actions. *Lancet* **i:** 658–659.

Plezia PM, Alberts DS, Kessler J, Aapro MS, Graham V & Surwit EA (1984) Immediate termination of intractable vomiting induced by cisplatin chemotherapy using an intensive five-drug antiemetic regimen. *Cancer Treatment Report* **68:** 1493–1495.

Reason JT & Brand JJ (1975) *Motion sickness.* New York: Academic Press.

Richardson BP, Engel G, Donatsch P & Stadler PA (1986) Identification of serotonin M-receptor subtypes and their specific blockades by a new class of drug. *Nature* **316:** 126–131.

Sallan SE, Zinberg NE & Frei E (1980) Antiemetic effect of delta-9-tetrahydrocannabinol and prochlorperazine. *New England Journal of Medicine* **302:** 135–138.
Saller R, Hellenbrecht D, Buhring M & Hess H (1986) Enhancement of the antiemetic action of metoclopramide against cisplatin-induced emesis by transdermal electrical nerve stimu-
Schultz-Delerieu K (1979) Metoclopramide. *Gastroenterology* **77:** 768–779.
Strum SB, McDermid JE, Pileggi J, Reich LP & Whittaker H (1984) Intravenous metoclopramide: prevention of chemotherapy-induced nausea and vomiting. *Cancer* **53:** 1432–1439.
Strum SB, McDermid JE & Liponi DF (1985) High-dose intravenous metoclopramide versus combination high-dose metoclopramide and intravenous dexamethasone in preventing cisplatin-induced nausea and emesis: a single-blind cross-over comparison of antiemetic efficacy. *Journal of Clinical Oncology* **3:** 245–248.
Swann IL, Thompson EN & Qureshi K (1979) Domperidone or metoclopramide in preventing chemotherapeutically-induced nausea and vomiting. *British Medical Journal* **2:** 1188.
Warrington PS, Allan SG, Cornbleet MA, Macpherson JS, Smyth JF & Leonard RCF (1986) Optimising antiemesis in cancer chemotherapy. Efficacy of continuous versus intermittent infusion of high-dose metoclopramide in emesis induced by cisplatin. *British Medical Journal* **293:** 1334–1337.
Wilcox PM, Fetting JH, Nettesheim KM & Abeloff MD (1982) Anticipatory vomiting in women receiving cyclophosphamide, methotrexate and 5-FU (CMF) adjuvant chemotherapy for breast carcinoma. *Cancer Treatment Report* **66:** 1601–1604.

5

Dysphagia

CLAUD F. B. REGNARD

> *Dysphagia*: Greek derivation: dys—combining form signifying difficult, painful, bad, disordered etc. phagein = to eat. (*Dorland's Illustrated Medical Dictionary*, 24th edition)
>
> 'I'm worried you know, about not being able to get things down—I've lost so much weight my bones are rattling together.' (Written by a patient with recurrent carcinoma of larynx.)

As children we were encouraged to eat to grow, to keep well and recover quickly from illness. As parents we worry when our children will not eat. No wonder then that anything that prevents eating is seen with fear by patients, relatives and care givers alike.

Dysphagia is difficulty in transferring solids or liquids from the oral cavity to the stomach. Although the journey is straightforward, the mechanism to achieve smooth and easy passage is complex. It requires an intact anatomy, normal mucosa, normal functioning of six cranial nerves and the brain-stem, the co-ordination of 34 skeletal muscles and co-ordination between striated muscle and smooth muscle (Table 1). Any disruption of this normal anatomy and physiology may result in dysphagia. An understanding of the normal process, followed by a careful assessment of the cause are therefore essential before treatment can start.

ANATOMY AND PHYSIOLOGY

Four phases can be differentiated in the journey from mouth to stomach (Logemann, 1983):

1. the oral preparatory phase;
2. the oral swallowing phase;
3. the pharyngeal phase;
4. the oesophageal phase.

In the first phase (Figure 1a) the food is mixed with saliva and prepared by chewing to break down larger particles. Individual preference will dictate the way the contents are moved within the mouth, but the common pattern is to keep the posterior tongue raised to protect the airway, whilst a food or liquid bolus is formed. Effective manipulation of the bolus depends upon co-ordination of the muscle groups and continuous interaction between oral sensory information and commands from reflex centres (such as the salivary

Table 1. The stages of swallowing.

Stage	Muscle group(s)	Cranial nerve supply	Time (s)	Voluntary control
Oral preparatory	mastication facial tongue	5 7 12	variable	Yes
Oral swallowing	facial soft palate tongue	7 5/10/11 12	1	Yes
Pharyngeal	pharyngeal	9/10/11	1	No
Oesophageal	striated (upper) smooth (lower) (middle mixed)	10	8–20	No

nucleus) and higher motor control centres in the cortex (Goldberg, 1976; Sessle, 1976).

In the oral swallowing phase (Figure 1b) the lips close to prevent leakage and the anterior tongue retracts and elevates. This elevation proceeds backwards in a wave and it is this voluntary action which pushes the bolus backwards to commence the next reflex phase.

The pharyngeal phase (Figure 1c) consists of several reflexes triggered by the bolus reaching the faucial arches and epiglottis (Figures 1a and 2b). The soft palate firstly rises to close the nasopharynx, followed by elevation of the larynx. The larynx is closed by the epiglottis and further protected by closure of the vocal cords and the cessation of breathing. The pharyngeal constrictors then move the bolus down by peristalsis. It takes the bolus less than a second to complete this stage of its journey, dividing either side of the epiglottis to reform above the oesophagus (Ardran and Kemp, 1951). Finally the cricopharyngeus muscle (Figure 2a) relaxes to allow material to pass into the oesophagus. This muscle can be considered as the upper oesophageal sphincter.

These complex actions are necessary since it is at the level of the pharynx that the airway crosses the alimentary tract. Above the pharynx the airway is ventral to the alimentary tract but it becomes dorsal below the pharynx. The pharynx is therefore a shared passage for air and food. Consequently these reflexes not only propel the bolus into the oesophagus but are also essential in protecting the airway (Storey, 1976).

The oesophageal phase (Figure 1d) carries the bolus on into the stomach at a rate of approximately $4\,cm \cdot s^{-1}$ (Gannong, 1977). The lower oesophagus is composed of smooth muscle with a low resting luminal pressure (0 mmHg) except at the gastro-oesophageal junction (30 mmHg) (Dodds, 1976). This area relaxes to allow the bolus to pass and functions as a lower oesophageal sphincter (Cohen and Harris, 1972).

Although initiating swallowing is a voluntary act, reflexes take over at an early stage in order to protect the airway. The neurological coordination is complex and involves the cortex, limbic system, basal ganglia, cerebellum

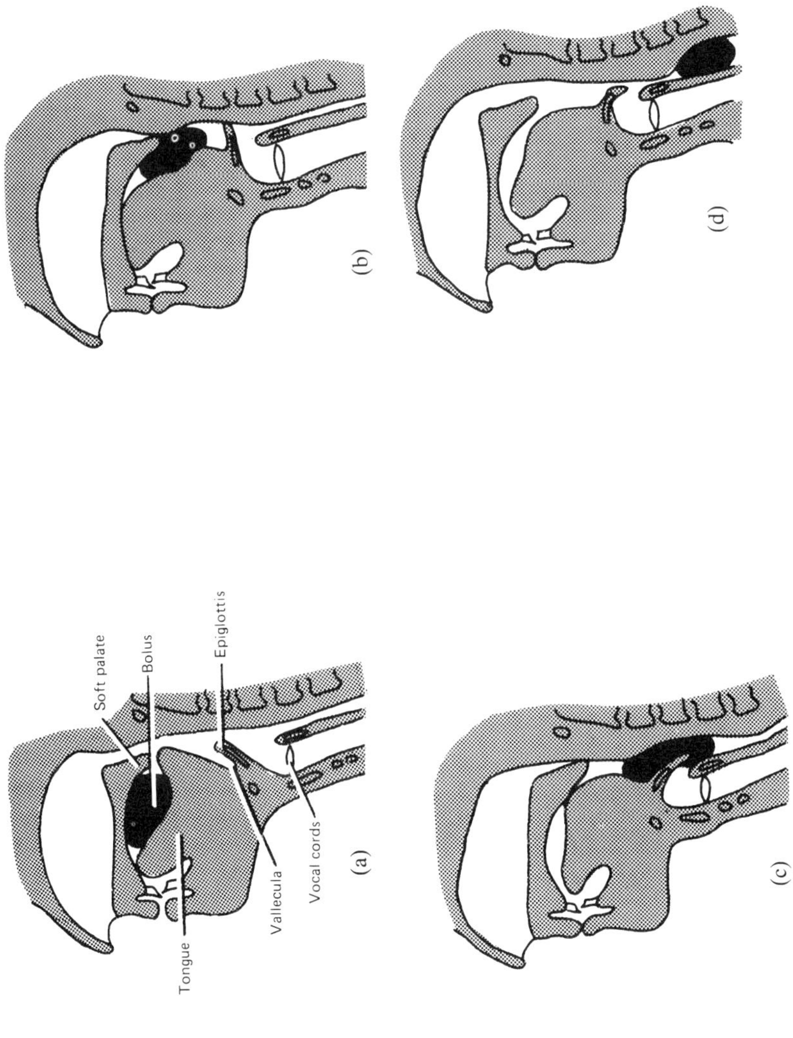

Figure 1. Four stages of swallowing can be distinguished on fluoroscopy: (a) the oral preparatory phase, (b) the oral swallowing phase, (c) the pharyngeal phase and (d) the oesophageal phase.

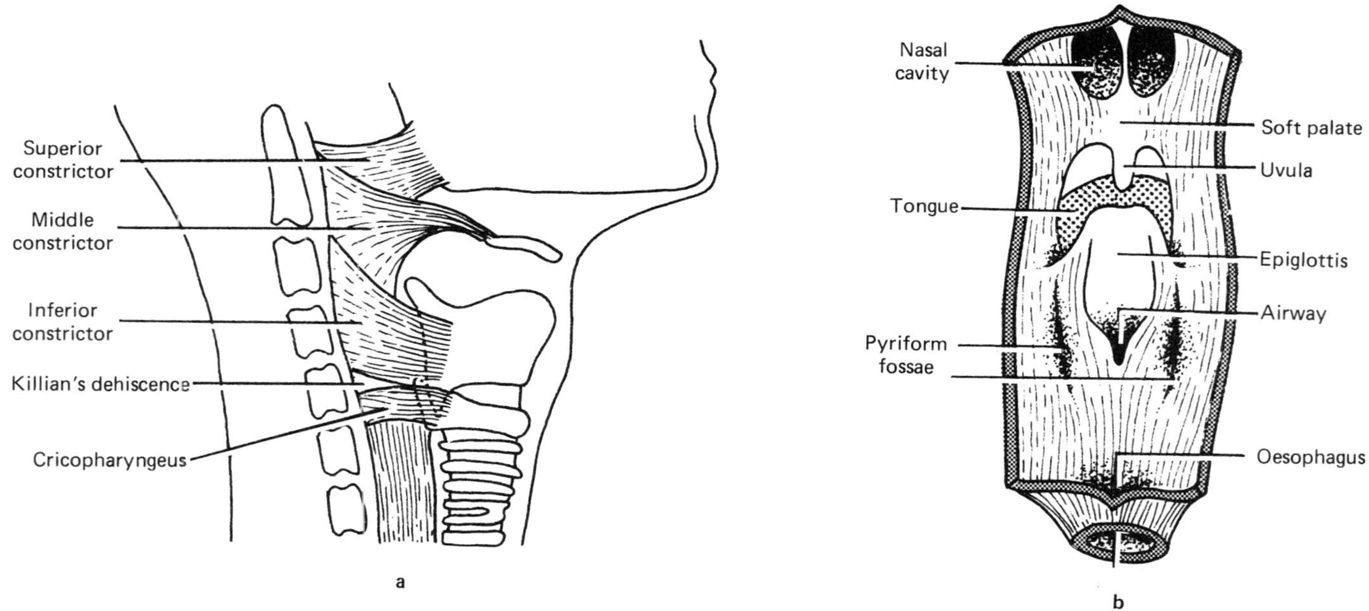

Figure 2. (a) Lateral view of the pharyngeal constrictors. (b) Anterior pharynx viewed through the opened posterior wall. Liquid food passes either side of the epiglottis into the pyriform fossae, before entering the oesophagus.

and brain-stem centres involved in respiration, salivation and motor function (Dellow, 1976). This complexity reflects the evolutionary necessity for respiration and nutrition, with respiration taking priority.

AETIOLOGY

In patients with cancer, dysphagia may be directly caused by the malignant process, by its treatment or may be a consequence of associated conditions (Table 2).

Malignancies will either alter function or cause an obstruction. Luminal and intramural growths in the oral cavity will tend to affect function. Tumours of the floor of the mouth may restrict tongue elevation and prevent adequate bolus manipulation. Lingual infiltration by tumour will have a similar effect, in addition to preventing backwards propulsion of the bolus, so failing to trigger the swallowing reflex. Inability to raise the posterior tongue may allow food to trickle into the pharynx and into an unprotected airway (Figure 3). Destruction of the upper gum or hard palate may cause nasal regurgitation. Loss of the soft palate and related structures such as the faucial pillars may cause aspiration in addition to nasal regurgitation. Pharyngeal infiltration by tumour may cause dysfunction if peristalsis is

Table 2. Causes of dysphagia related to cancer.

Caused by cancer	*Caused by treatment*
Luminal: • oral • pharyngeal • oesophageal	Surgery: • loss or alteration of structure • fibrosis • fistula formation • motor/sensory loss
Intramural: • lingual infiltration • pharyngo-oesophageal infiltration	Post radiation: • reduced saliva • mucosal inflammation • fibrosis, osteoradionecrosis
Extramural: • mediastinal nodes or tumour • parapharyngeal tumours	Post chemotherapy: • mucosal ulceration, herpes zoster
Neurological: • metastatic—upper motor neurone (cerebral tumour or metastases) —lower motor neurone (brain-stem tumours or metastases, perineural spread)	*Associated with debility* Oral, pharyngeal or oesophageal candidosis Herpes simplex Excessive drowsiness and disinterest Extreme weakness
• non metastatic—neuromuscular paraneoplastic syndromes	*Concurrent causes* Oesophageal spasm (anxiety, drugs) Benign oesophageal stricture (reflux, drugs) Dry mouth (anxiety, drugs, infection) Pain (mucosal inflammation or infection, soft tissue infection, dental caries)
Pain (soft tissue infiltration, bone invasion, perineural spread)	

Adapted from Twycross RG and Lack SA (1986), with permission.

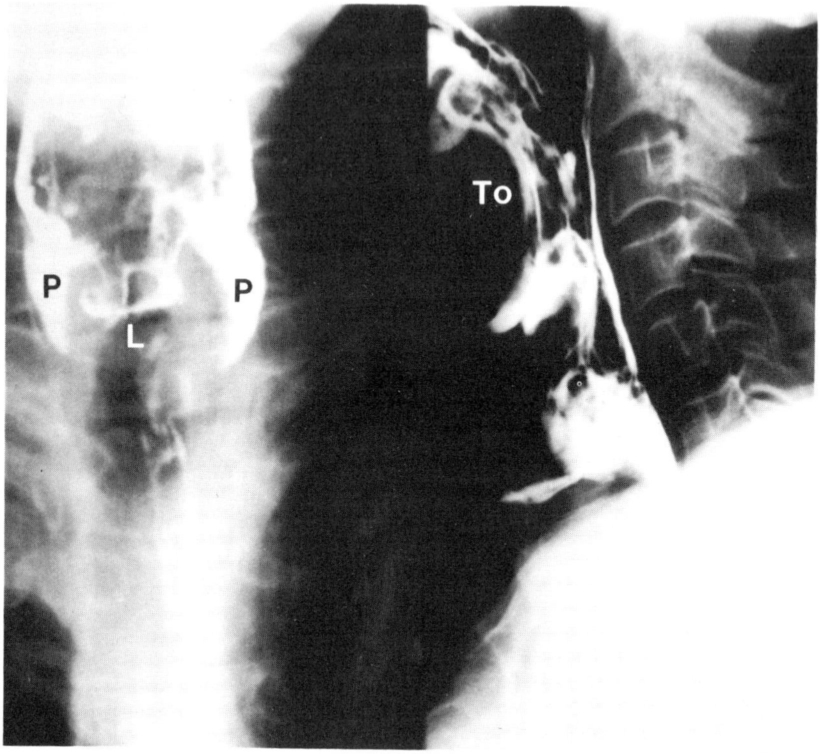

Figure 3. Anteroposterior and lateral views of a barium swallow in a patient with poor lingual movement caused by lingual infiltration with a squamous cell carcinoma of the base of the tongue. Barium is seen trickling over the posterior tongue (To) and into the pyriform fossae (P) with spilling of barium into the entrance of the larynx (L).

reduced, or obstruction if the cricopharyngeus muscle is unable to relax and allow the bolus to pass.

Tumours of the lower pharynx are often silent at first but as they enlarge will cause obstruction with progressive dysphagia. Pharyngeal and laryngeal sensory loss due to tumour involvement of the superior laryngeal nerve will cause 'silent' aspiration. Luminal growths of the pharynx or oesophagus tend to cause obstruction (Figure 4). Food will collect proximally and may eventually spill over into an unprotected airway (Figure 5). Extramural compression of the pharynx by a parapharyngeal tumour, or of the oesophagus by mediastinal nodes or tumour will have the same effect.

Neurological sequelae tend to be functional. Cerebral metastases or tumours may result in motor dysfunction, especially of the tongue and lips, which will affect the oral phases. Unilateral lesions will result in food collecting on the paralysed side and increase oral transit time. Analysis of swallowing problems in stroke patients shows that hemisphere lesions can cause reduced lingual control, a delayed swallowing reflex and reduced

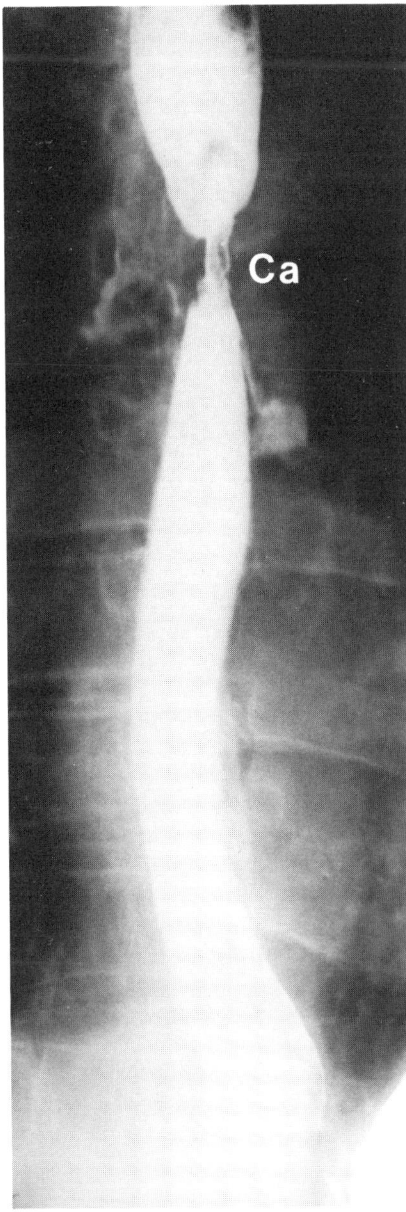

Figure 4. Anteroposterior view of a barium swallow showing obstruction due to a carcinoma of the middle oesophagus (Ca).

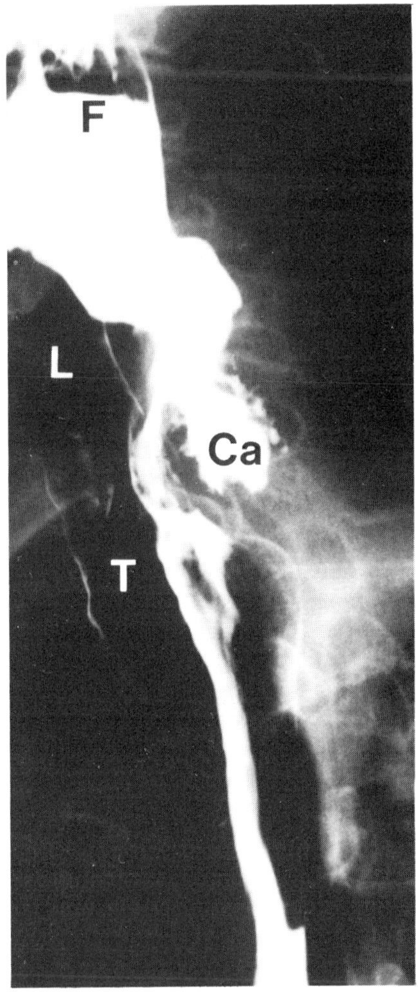

Figure 5. Lateral view of barium swallow showing an ulcerating squamous cell carcinoma of the upper oesophagus (Ca) with poor pharyngeal emptying demonstrated by the presence of a fluid level in the pharynx (F). Laryngeal (L) and tracheal (T) aspiration of barium can be seen.

pharyngeal peristalsis (Veis and Logemann, 1985). Cranial nerves may be damaged by tumours of the posterior nasal space or soft palate infiltrating along the skull base. The lower cranial nerves and their nuclei may be damaged by brain-stem metastases or tumours. The closeness of these nuclei to each other and to motor, sensory and other pathways can produce complex results (Table 3). Perineural invasion of cranial nerves by tumour has been clearly shown by Carter et al (1982) in patients with squamous carcinoma of the head and neck. In this series the overall frequency of perineural spread was 44% at the time of surgery but rose to 88% at post mortem. The 5th and 9th cranial nerves were most commonly involved. Although sensory changes predominated, dysphagia was also due to a variable combination of perineural invasion of one or more cranial nerves and splinting of the pharynx by fibrosis and tumour.

Occasionally dysphagia results from non-metastatic (paraneoplastic) effects of tumours. The myasthenic–myopathic syndrome is usually associated with oat-cell carcinoma of the bronchus. Like myasthenia gravis there is proximal muscle weakness which may involve swallowing. In contrast to myasthenia, muscle power can increase after brief exercise, tendon reflexes are depressed or absent and neostigmine is only partly effective in temporarily reversing the weakness. Polymyositis may cause dysphagia through oesophageal dysfunction and is classically associated with both carcinoma and lymphoma, although this association is now being challenged. Other unusual non-metastatic effects include cerebellar dysfunction associated with carcinoma of ovary, breast or lung.

Pain that is precipitated or worsened by swallowing movements will result in dysphagia. The pain may be due to mucosal changes caused by infection, radiotherapy or chemotherapy. Infiltration by tumour into muscle, soft tissues, the laryngeal skeleton or bone, will itself be painful. Pain occurs in over 50% of head and neck cancer patients (Aird et al, 1983) with a higher proportion developing pain in cancers involving the lower pharynx and submandibular region (Robertson and Hornibrook, 1982). The pain can be

Table 3. Effects of brain-stem damage on swallowing.

Level with structures that may be involved	Effect on swallowing	Other possible effects
Pons (7th nerve, 6th nucleus, 5th nucleus, motor and sensory long tracts)	Abnormal oral phase (ipsilateral facial paralysis, sensory loss and paralysis of masticatory muscles)	Contralateral hemiplegia, impaired conjugate gaze to side of lesion, contralateral sensory loss of body
Medulla (vestibular nuclei, 5th nucleus and tract, reticular formation, nucleus ambiguous, descending autonomic fibres, 9–12th nuclei, motor and sensory long tracts)	Abnormal preparatory phase (masticatory paralysis, ipsilateral tongue paralysis and wasting) Abnormal swallowing reflex with aspiration (ipsilateral sensory loss)	Tetraplegia, contralateral hemi- or monoplegia, hoarseness, hiccups, vertigo, vomiting, ipsilateral cerebellar signs, ipsilateral Horner's syndrome

severe with a combination of causes: small fascial compartments allowing little room for tumour expansion, perineural invasion by tumour (Carter et al, 1982), bone invasion and tissue infection.

Surgery may cause dysphagia by anatomical distortion at operation or during scar formation, or by disrupting the nerves mediating the complex reflex arcs (Table 4). Oedema in the immediate postoperative period will compromise swallowing but is usually temporary. Resection of less than 50% of the tongue may not cause serious swallowing problems if no other structures are involved (Conley, 1960). Less extensive surgery, however, can still cause significant problems if tongue mobility is reduced by pro-

Table 4. Effects of surgery on swallowing.

Cause	Effect on swallowing	Consequence
Glossectomy (partial or complete), lingual–labial closures, floor of mouth resections, tongue flap repairs	Abnormal preparatory phase, poor triggering of swallowing reflex	Poor bolus formation and control, drooling, collection of food in lateral sulci and on hard palate, delayed transit, aspiration
Buccal flaps	Reduced buccal tension	Collection of food in lateral sulci, drooling
Mandibular resection	Misalignment of teeth	Less effective mastication and bolus formation
Submental resections	Reduced laryngeal elevation with poor airway protection	Aspiration
Hemilaryngectomy or supraglottic laryngectomy	Delayed swallowing reflex, reduced laryngeal closure (especially if arytenoid cartilage removed), reduced glottic protection if tongue base removed, reduced pharyngeal peristalsis if pharyngeal resection occurs	Delayed oral and pharyngeal transit, aspiration
Total laryngectomy	Scarring of base of tongue or pharynx, cricopharyngeal spasm, abnormal oesophageal motility	Pharyngeal occlusion or stricture, aspiration
Disruption of motor pathways (5, 7, 9–12)	Inefficient swallowing phases	Delayed transit times, nasal regurgitation
Disruption of sensory pathways (5, 9, 10)	Inefficient mastication, swallowing reflex not triggered, reduced laryngeal sensation	Poor bolus formation and control, collection of food in lateral sulci, delayed oral transit, 'silent' aspiration
Infection (post-operative)	Pain, tracheo-oesophageal fistula	Painful swallowing, aspiration
	Pharyngo-cutaneous fistula	Leakage of saliva, food

cedures such as tongue flap repairs or tongue-to-lip closures (Logemann and Bytell, 1979). These will seriously affect the oral preparatory phase and delay triggering of the swallowing reflex (Logemann, 1983). Floor of mouth resections may reduce lingual function and reduce triggering of the swallowing reflex if the faucial arches are involved. Hemilaryngectomy will rarely cause swallowing problems if the epiglottis is preserved, unlike a unilateral supraglottic laryngectomy which is more likely to result in a chronic swallowing disability (Weaver and Fleming, 1978). Total laryngectomy may be followed by stricture formation, or abnormal motility of the cricopharyngeus and oesophagus (Duranceau et al, 1976). With resections of the cervical oesophagus, continuity can be restored using skin flaps, or by visceral transposition using the stomach (Harrison et al, 1981) or ascending colon. Dysphagia is more likely with skin flap reconstructions. Finally, postoperative fibrosis may cause partial obstruction of the pharynx or oesophagus, or restrict laryngeal elevation which is an important component of airway protection.

Radiotherapy involving the oral cavity may affect swallowing in several ways (Ritchie et al, 1985). Salivary flow is reduced and the resultant dry mouth (xerostomia) will affect the oral and pharyngeal phases of swallowing. It appears during the course of treatment and may last several months or more. Removal of the protective effect of saliva on the teeth is probably why severe caries is more prevalent after oral radiotherapy, and the resultant pain may disturb the oral preparatory phase. Consequently prophylactic dental clearance may be performed prior to treatment. Mucosal inflammation (mucositis), which is painful, appears during therapy but usually resolves 2–3 weeks after treatment has stopped. *Candida albicans* occurs more frequently in irradiated head and neck cancer patients (Silverman et al, 1984). Uncommon effects of radiotherapy are osteoradionecrosis of the jaw which will cause misalignment, and trismus due to radiation-induced fibrosis of muscle tissue and the temporomandibular joint.

Chemotherapy may also cause mucositis, the severity reflecting the extent of bone marrow suppression (Lockhart and Sonis, 1979). Antimetabolites, antibiotics and plant alkaloids all have oral effects, but in one study the agents most frequently associated with oral problems were doxorubicin hydrochloride, cyclophosphamide, vincristine sulphate and methotrexate (Sonis et al, 1978). The subsequent immunosuppression may also result in re-activation of herpes zoster. This virus may infect the mandibular or maxillary branches of the trigeminal nerve causing a painful oral preparatory phase.

General debility from any cause related to the cancer or its treatment may result in re-activation of the herpes simplex virus or opportunistic infection by *Candida*. Herpes simplex, like herpes zoster, may infect the maxillary and mandibular branches of the trigeminal nerve. Painful, shallow aphthous ulcers, which affect the oral preparatory phase of swallowing, are the result. Most overt candidosis is probably the result of an overgrowth of *Candida* following a reduction in host immunity. *Candida* may affect the mouth, pharynx and oesophagus. Oral candidosis may present with a thin red mucosa, angular chelitis, pale patches of chronically infected epithelium, or

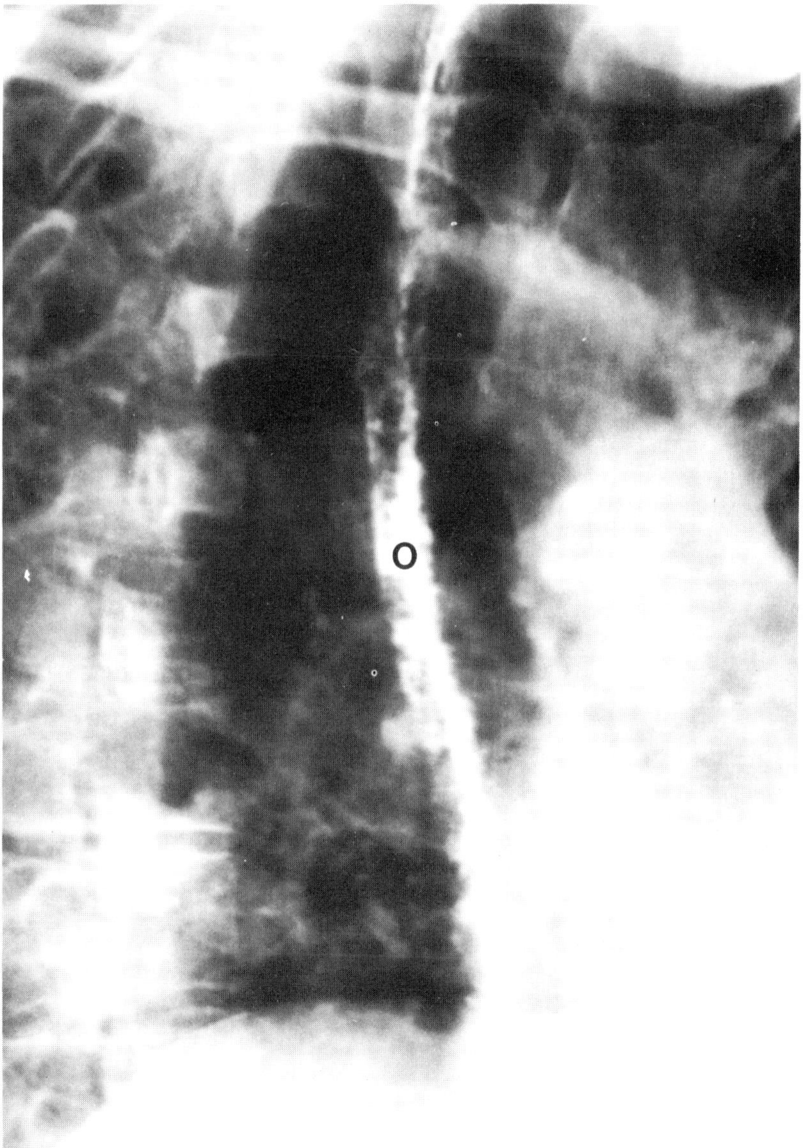

Figure 6. Barium swallow showing the ragged appearance of an oesophagus heavily overgrown with *Candida* (O). This appearance may also be caused by ulceration due to herpes simplex or cytomegalovirus infection.

the classical white patches which leave an erythematous area when rubbed away (Gilmour and Chustecki, 1984). Pharyngeal or oesophageal candidosis present with painful dysphagia (odynophagia), and in the oesophagus the pain may radiate to retrosternal, paravertebral or intrascapular regions. Oesophageal candidosis may also present with minor haematemesis. Oral

Candida is found in only 50% of patients with oesophageal candidosis (Trier and Bjorkman, 1984). The appearances of ulceration on barium swallow are characteristic (Figure 6) and can also be caused by herpes simplex or cytomegalovirus infection.

Excessive drowsiness, disinterest and weakness will result in a poor oral preparatory phase with leakage of food from the mouth, drooling, and possibly aspiration due to poor triggering of the swallowing reflex.

Anxiety and emotional stress increase lower oesophageal pressure (Rogers et al, 1980) and can cause cricopharyngeal spasm, both of which may result in dysphagia. Drugs may affect swallowing in a variety of ways (Table 5): by reducing salivary secretions, by increasing lower oesophageal tone, causing reflux by decreasing lower oesophageal tone, by producing extrapyramidal effects, by reducing oral sensation, or by mucosal irritation.

FREQUENCY

The frequency of dysphagia in patients with head and neck cancer was 38% in the series by Aird et al (1983). Robertson and Hornibrook (1982) found that 43% of their series presented with dysphagia, with 83% eventually suffering from dysphagia. This second study also looked at the frequency at different sites of the oropharynx, finding that the tumour site most commonly associated with dysphagia was the post-cricoid region (Figure 7).

Table 5. Effect of drugs on swallowing.

Drug	Possible effect on swallowing	Consequence
Anticholinergic e.g. atropine, hyoscine hydrobromide, tricyclic antidepressants, chlorpromazine, prochlorperazine	Reduced salivary secretions	Delayed oral transit time
	Reduced lower oesophageal tone	Reflux oesophagitis
	Extrapyramidal symptoms	Disordered oral preparatory phase
Nicotine, diazepam, theophylline, glyceryl trinitrate	Reduced lower oesophageal tone	Reflux oesophagitis
Metoclopramide hydrochloride, domperidone	Increased lower oesophageal tone	Lower oesophageal hold-up
Emepronium bromide	Mucosal ulceration	Painful swallowing
Dopamine antagonists (e.g. haloperidol	Extrapyramidal symptoms	Disordered oral preparatory phase
Lignocaine, benzydamine	Local anaesthesia	Reduced oral sensation
Nitrazepam	Delayed cricopharyngeal relaxation	Drooling, aspiration
Chlormethiazole edisylate	Abnormal oesophageal co-ordination	Aspiration

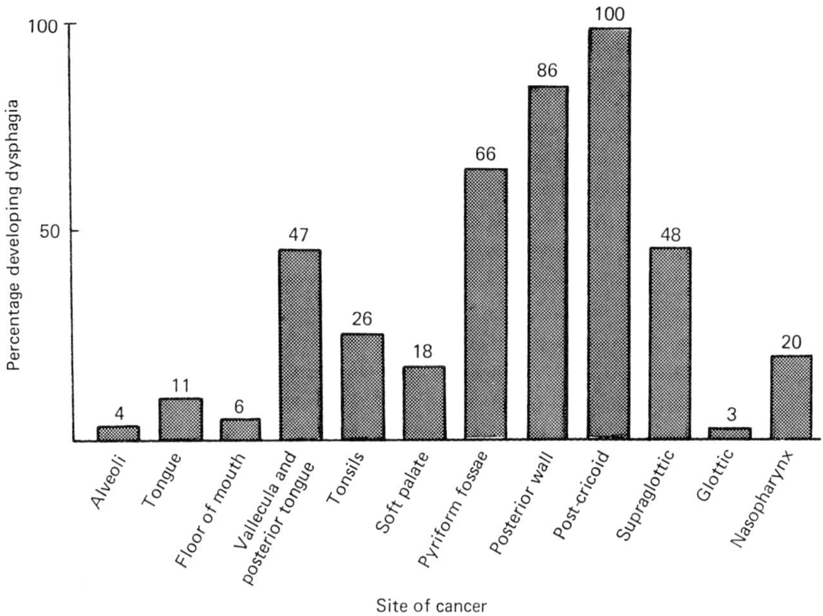

Figure 7. Frequency of dysphagia for tumours in different sites of the oropharynx. (Adapted from data in Robertson and Hornibrook, 1982.)

EVALUATION

A basic evaluation can be carried out by the clinician, but further important information and helpful advice should be sought from the speech therapist and radiologist.

History

Patients, families and nurses can provide much useful information. The patient's description of swallowing is remarkably accurate. In one series of 1000 patients, localization by the patient corresponded to the anatomical site of the problem in 99.2% of cases (Logemann, 1983). Occasionally patients deny a problem which has already been identified by family or nurses, particularly in patients with neurological disorders. The history and any observed difficulty in handling food at different stages of swallowing will suggest the level of the abnormality (Table 6). Difficulties with certain food consistencies may indicate a particular problem but are not specific for that problem. Symptoms suggesting aspiration are important and include choking or coughing, a 'gargle' type voice, copious expectoration or a history of chest infections. Troublesome secretions are more likely in patients with an impaired cough reflex and result from irritation of the smaller airways by aspirated material.

Other important symptoms are mouth odour (suggesting oral or pharyngeal infection), pain on swallowing, voice changes, or dyspnoea. The site and radiation of pain may suggest the level of the problem. For example, sharp, intermittent pain referred to the ear (via the vagus) may suggest a tumour of the pyriform fossae, base of tongue, vallecula, or suggest oesophageal compression by a bronchial carcinoma. Pain on swallowing suggests inflammation, infection or malignant invasion. Lower pharyngeal tumours rarely produce hoarseness, and vallecular tumours produce voice changes only at a late stage, producing a voice akin to having a hot potato in the mouth. Tumours of the lower pharynx and oesophagus may cause hoarseness by damaging the recurrent laryngeal nerve, producing a 'breathy' voice. Stridor and dyspnoea can be the result of supraglottic tumours. Finally information about medication may suggest a cause (see Table 5) and the exact nature of previous surgery involving the head, neck and upper gastro-intestinal tract should be noted (see Table 4).

Examination

Useful information on the first three phases of swallowing can be obtained from an examination by the clinician, but more detailed information will be obtained by requesting the help of a speech therapist with experience in treating swallowing disorders.

The face should be observed for signs of weakness, evidence of drooling or leakage of food. The presence of stridor should be noted. During chewing, misalignment of the jaw may be apparent, as may facial weakness, with bulging of one cheek. Lip closure during chewing is observed and lip function can be further checked by rapidly repeating a syllable such as 'pa'. The mouth should be inspected for signs of food collecting on the palate or lateral sulci. The condition of the teeth should be noted and the mucosa checked for dryness, inflammation or signs of infection.

Movement of the anterior tongue can be observed while the patient is asked to pass the tongue tip along the occlusive surfaces of upper and lower teeth. Movement of the posterior tongue can be checked by rapidly repeating the syllable 'ka'. An estimate of the strength of the tongue can be made by placing a gloved finger on the tongue and asking the patient to push the finger against the hard palate. Sensation of the oral mucosa can be assessed using a cold laryngeal mirror. The vallecula (see Figure 1a) and pyriform fossae (see Figure 2b) should be inspected with a laryngeal mirror for evidence of food debris which would suggest an incomplete swallowing reflex with the risk of aspiration. The same instrument can be used to observe the palatal reflex by touching the soft palate which should then elevate. The gag reflex is elicited by touching the posterior pharyngeal wall or the base of the tongue when both the pharynx and soft palate should contract strongly. The presence or absence of the gag reflex, however, is not necessarily an indication of the patient's ability to swallow (Logemann, 1983). Abnormal laryngeal function is suggested by dysphonia or difficulty coughing and advice should be sought from an ENT surgeon and speech therapist for further assessment.

A test swallow can provide further useful information. The material to swallow will depend on the assessment so far. For example, those with delayed swallowing reflexes or symptoms of aspiration will do better with soft material such as mashed potatoes. The patient may suggest which consistencies he or she finds easiest to swallow. It is also important to know which head positions a patient prefers (see Table 6). A patient who keeps his head down throughout taking food and swallowing is widening the vallecular space to protect the airway further, suggesting poor laryngeal closure. A patient who tilts the head backwards on swallowing may be compensating for poor tongue control.

Before swallowing it is helpful if the clinician places the index finger in the submandibular region to feel tongue movement, with the other fingers over the larynx. On swallowing it will then be possible to assess roughly oral transit time between the first tongue movement and last laryngeal movement. Times of more than one second are abnormal. If coughing or choking occurs it should be noted whether this is before, during or after swallowing (see Table 6). On completion of swallowing the patient should be asked to speak, since some patients aspirate silently and, although not coughing or choking, will have a 'gargle' quality to their voice.

Investigation

The examination may uncover the cause of dysphagia, especially in the oral preparatory phase. Accurate assessment of the remaining phases is best done radiologically. This is particularly important with aspiration since in one study aspiration was correctly diagnosed by clinical examination in only approximately 60% of cases (Logemann, 1983). One to two ml of liquid barium are used initially and a single film taken approximately 2 s after commencing the oral swallowing phase. Further films of the pharynx should be taken up to 30 s after the swallow to exclude aspiration (Logemann, 1985). Such single films may show aspiration clearly (see Figures 3 and 5). If no aspiration is present larger volumes of barium can be swallowed which may show more distal obstructions (see Figure 4) or oesophageal abnormalities (see Figure 6). Aspiration, an abnormal pharyngeal phase or disordered oesophageal motility are best assessed by cine- or video-fluoroscopy (Logemann and Bytell, 1979; Logemann, 1983; Ott et al, 1986). Pharyngoscopy and direct laryngoscopy may be necessary to assess local lesions by observation and biopsy. Endoscopy will assess oesophageal lesions, but cannot assess oesophageal motility. This can be assessed using manometry which measures intra-luminal pressure at different levels of the oesophagus (Dodds, 1976), but will have a limited application in patients with advanced cancer.

MANAGEMENT

Many of the early treatment decisions in dysphagia can be made by the clinician and nurse (Figure 8). For other treatment options, however, the help and advice of a speech therapist with an interest in swallowing disorders is invaluable.

Table 6. Evaluation of dysphagia.

Information provided	Possible interpretation(s)
Leakage from mouth, drooling	Poor lip closure, reduced lip sensation, abnormal tongue movement or reduced/absent swallowing reflex
Bites cheeks or tongue	Reduced lip or tongue sensation
Frequent nasal regurgitation	Palatal dysfunction
Food collecting:	
• in mouth	Poor lip, buccal or tongue control
• in vallecula/pyriform fossae	Reduced/absent swallowing reflex
Patient washes food down with a drink, or pushes food in with finger Patient tilts head down on taking in food, then backwards on swallowing	Reduced tongue control
Patient keeps head down throughout swallowing	Delayed swallowing reflex or poor laryngeal closure
Difficulty with solids:	
• in triggering swallowing	Poor tongue control
• food 'sticks': at upper neck	Hold up in upper/mid-pharynx
at lower neck	Lower-pharyngeal obstruction, cricopharyngeus muscle dysfunction, or upper-oesophageal obstruction
over sternum	Mid-oesophageal hold-up
epigastrium	Lower-oesophageal hold-up
• lack of awareness of where food is during swallowing	Pharyngeal sensory loss
Difficulty with liquids	Poor tongue control, reduced/absent swallowing reflex, severe obstruction, muscular inco-ordination, soft palate paralysis or fixation
Coughing, choking:	Aspiration due to:
• before swallowing	• poor tongue control or delayed/absent swallowing reflex
• during swallowing	• reduced airway protection
• after swallowing	• reduced pharyngeal emptying, reduced laryngeal elevation, cricopharyngeus dysfunction, pharyngeal or oesophageal obstruction or tracheo-oesophageal fistula
'Gargle' type voice, copious expectorations, recurrent fever and chest infections	Aspiration
Pain on swallowing	Ulceration/inflammation (infection, malignant invasion, irradiation, drugs)

The need for hydration and feeding

It is important to decide the need for drink and food at the outset. It is natural that relatives and staff should wish to feed a patient, since food and particularly fluid are seen as the minimum requirements for sustaining life. For much of a patient's life there is no conflict. In the last days, however,

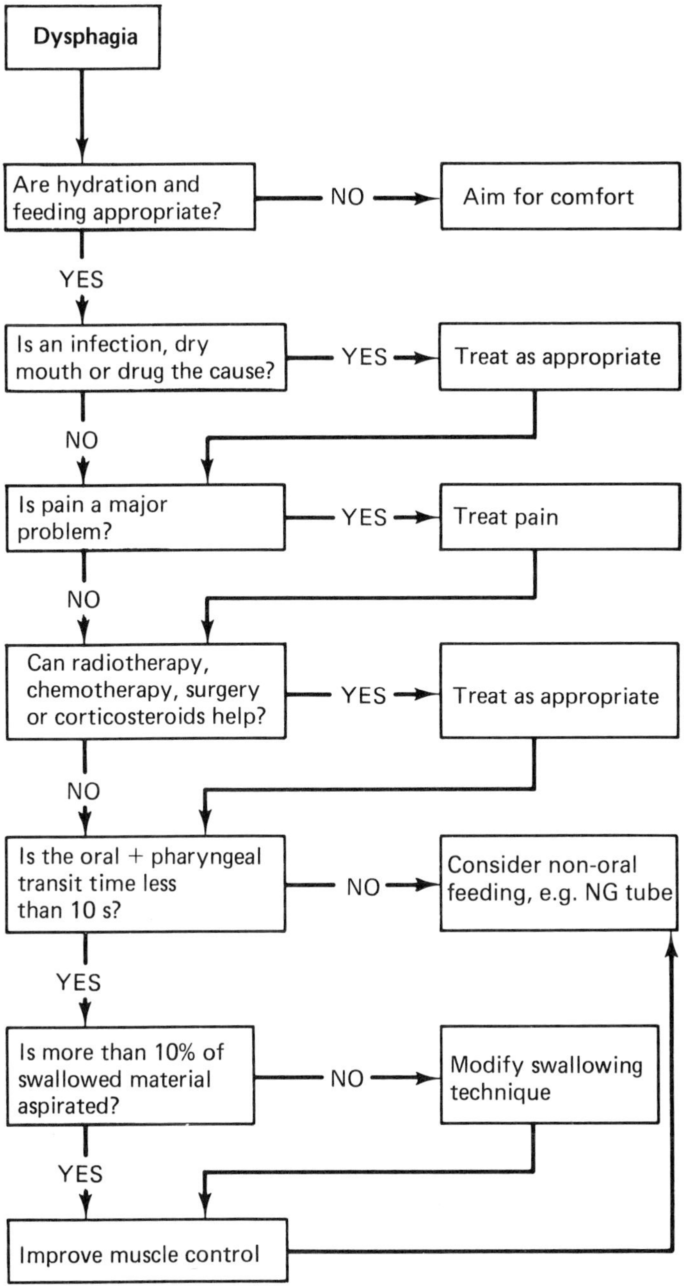

Figure 8. Flow diagram in the management of dysphagia. NG = nasogastric.

there is danger that the need to sustain life overrides the patient's need for comfort. Eating for pleasure and for energy become separated as the patient deteriorates. In the last hours and days energy requirements are usually so low and anorexia so complete that feeding is unnecessary. As for dehydration, there is no evidence that the symptoms of experimental water deprivation or hyponatraemia are seen in patients with advanced cancer who are dehydrated (Billings, 1985). Indeed, intravenous hydration can be distressing (Editorial, 1986) and in very ill patients at the end of their lives dehydration can actually improve comfort (Twycross and Lack, 1986). Decreased urinary output reduces the need for catheterization, and troublesome bronchial secretions lessen. Regurgitation of swallowed saliva and secretions from oesophageal obstructions will also reduce. Neuromuscular irritability may be seen in marked dehydration, causing muscular jerks and restlessness. If troublesome these will settle with titrated doses of oral or rectal diazepam. A dry mouth can be treated with local measures (see below). The consequence is a peaceful terminal phase without recourse to intravenous hydration and tube-feeding.

Infections, dry mouths and drugs

Candida often responds to topical antifungals such as nystatin, amphotericin or miconazole. If dentures are worn these must be cleaned separately since *Candida* can live relatively protected on their surface. Commercial denture soaking agents can culture *Candida* while weak chlorine-releasing solutions such as diluted Milton (sodium hypochlorite) are antifungal. If the dentures contain metal they may be damaged by a chlorine-releasing solution and should be brushed with an antifungal.

Alternatively an antifungal such as ketoconazole can be given systemically. Ketoconazole has three advantages over nystatin: it can be given in a single daily dose of 200 mg for 7 days, at this dose it is currently cheaper than 2 ml nystatin 4-hourly, and the need to clean dentures is lessened. Symptoms usually settle in 2–3 days. Serious side-effects are rare with ketoconazole (Hay, 1985) and an incidence of potentially serious hepatic injury of 1 in 15 000 exposed individuals (Lewis et al, 1984) should not preclude its use in advanced cancer.

Prophylactic antifungals do not reduce the incidence of positive mouth swabs (Finlay, 1986), but in a few patients long-term therapy may be necessary to prevent symptoms returning. Most candidosis appears to be due to an overgrowth of existing *Candida* although cross infection has been reported as occurring via carers' hands (Burnie et al, 1985a) but it does not appear to occur via cups and cutlery. Since chlorhexidine is not effective for hand washing, fungicidal disinfectants such as povidone-iodine should be used (Burnie et al, 1985b).

Herpes zoster infection may respond to oral acyclovir 200 mg five times daily for 5 days. Oral or topical acyclovir can be used in herpes simplex infections. Topical applications which have been shown to speed healing of oral herpes simplex ulcers include tetracycline as a mouthwash, chlorhexidine gluconate or acetate, and corticosteroids such as betamethasone, triamcinolone or hydrocortisone. Steroids can be mixed with Orabase (carmellose sodium) and applied to local lesions while multiple ulcers are best treated with a tetracycline mouthwash 250 mg 8-hourly.

A dry mouth will respond to increased oral intake if this is appropriate and if dehydration is the cause. In other situations local measures can be effective.

Regular mouth care is essential. In addition, humidifying the room air reduces mucosal dehydration and a petroleum jelly on the lips prevents cracking. Artificial salivas contain methylcellulose with lemon essence or other additives for taste. Their use appears attractive but they cannot replace natural saliva and some patients complain of an oily taste. To be effective artificial salivas need to be given hourly either via a dropper or spray. Glycerol has a dehydrating effect on the mucosa and is best avoided. Water is often more effective, especially ice-cold or frozen. Crushed ice, frozen tonic water or frozen orange juice are easy to chew and suck. An alternative is to increase salivation by sucking ascorbic acid tablets or sharp sweets. Pineapple chunks are easily chewed and contain a proteolytic enzyme, ananase, which helps keep the mouth clean. Fresh pineapple tends to be too sharp to taste and tinned pineapple is often preferred. It is perhaps best to choose the unsweetened variety, although there is no evidence that their sugar content predisposes to *Candida*.

Alternative drugs may have to be used, such as changing from amitriptyline hydrochloride to an antidepressant with fewer anticholinergic adverse effects such as mianserin hydrochloride. Prochlorperazine is a commonly used anti-emetic which can cause a dry mouth, and a satisfactory alternative for chemically-induced nausea and vomiting is low-dose haloperidol (1.5–3 mg at night), which is unlikely to cause this problem. It is important that patients take tablets with at least 150 ml water, ideally sitting up, otherwise tablets may stick in the oesophagus. Lodged tablets may cause local ulceration, particularly with drugs such as emepronium bromide.

Pain

Pain caused by malignant infiltration of soft tissues will usually respond to regular, titrated oral doses of either a weak opioid (dihydrocodeine tartrate, co-proxamol) or a strong opioid (morphine, diamorphine hydrochloride) (Regnard and Davies, 1986). The analgesic is chosen not on the basis of pain severity but on the patient's response. If a patient is not controlled on a non-opioid, a weak opioid is the next step. If maximum doses of a weak opioid (e.g. 60 mg dihydrocodeine 4-hourly) do not control the pain then a strong opioid is the next logical step. There is no maximum dose for oral morphine, the median dose being 20 mg 4-hourly, although the median 4-hourly dose for head and neck cancer patients is 30 mg. Most patients are controlled on 100 mg 4-hourly or less. There is no evidence that cancer patients on oral morphine are troubled with psychological dependence. Contrary to popular belief, tolerance to pain relief is slow to develop and probably self-limiting. In contrast, tolerance to sedation is rapid (5–7 days) and prophylactic anti-emetics such as haloperidol 1.5–3 mg at night can usually be stopped ten days after starting oral morphine. There is no tolerance to constipation and prophylactic laxatives should always be given.

Patients with pain due to involvement of bone will benefit from the addition of a non-steroidal anti-inflammatory drug. Where pain is caused by pressure effects within a tight fascial compartment, corticosteroids will reduce peri-tumour oedema with resultant pain relief. The same principle can be used for pain caused by peri-neural invasion by tumour. A suitable regimen is dexamethasone 8–16 mg daily on a reducing dosage.

Mucosal inflammation or ulceration due to infection, radiotherapy or chemotherapy is often painful. Topical analgesics for oral soreness can be helpful. Diphenhydramine hydrochloride is an antihistamine present in Benadryl and Histergan which can be used alone or mixed with Kaopectate (light kaolin) or Orabase to allow it to adhere to the mucosa. Drowsiness can occur if large amounts are swallowed. Choline salicylate gel (Bonjela, Teejel) is analgesic but can be painful on initial application. Benzydamine hydrochloride is a non-steroidal anti-inflammatory drug. Used as a mouthwash (Difflam) it has a mild local anaesthetic action in the mouth and is particularly useful in radiation-induced mucositis (Kim et al, 1985). Local anaesthetics such as lignocaine in gels or sprays are effective but the resultant numbness can severely compromise swallowing. Maximum dose recommendations for lignocaine vary depending on the source, but a maximum 600 mg daily is a guide, although this should be reduced if there is widespread ulceration.

Oesophagitis due to radiation will be eased by oxethazaine, a local anaesthetic which is contained in Mucaine, in doses of 10–15 ml Mucaine before meals and at bedtime. Radiation oesophagitis has also been shown to respond to the prophylactic administration of a non-steroidal anti-inflammatory drug (Nicolopoulos et al, 1985).

Radiotherapy, chemotherapy, surgery and corticosteroids

Many patients who presented with primary malignancies causing dysphagia will have been treated by irradiation, chemotherapy, surgical resection or a combination, often with cure as the aim. Patients with recurrent disease or who present with advanced disease, however, may still benefit from one or more of these treatment modalities.

Recurrent squamous carcinoma of the head and neck can be palliated with radiotherapy as long as the tissues to be irradiated have received previous doses below normal tissue tolerance. Even in patients who have previously received radical radiotherapy transient palliation can sometimes be achieved with small, localized fields or radioactive implants. Chemotherapy appears to offer little advantage to such patients since clinical tumour regressions often require combination regimens with significant side-effects and without prolongation of life. Radical surgery can be helpful in selected cases with severe dysphagia (Harrison et al, 1981), while simpler techniques can be useful such as injecting Teflon into a paralysed vocal cord to improve laryngeal protection. Surgery will also have a place in non-oral feeding (see below), but for many patients with advanced, recurrent disease surgery appears to have little palliative value (Pittam, 1982).

Dysphagia due to oesophageal carcinoma is a difficult problem. It can sometimes be usefully palliated by external radiotherapy in patients who have not been previously irradiated. Single-dose intra-oesophageal irradiation using the 'Selectron' relieved dysphagia due to advanced oesophageal carcinoma in up to 70% of patients for as long as 50 weeks, and the method was suggested as an alternative to intubation (Rowland and Pagliero, 1985). Irradiation may be helpful in lower oesophageal dysphagia due to gastric carcinoma (Mantell, 1982). Extrinsic pressure from malignant lymphoma generally responds well to radiotherapy or chemotherapy, and pressure from a bronchial carcinoma, although less radiosensitive, may be helped by radiotherapy. Chemotherapy of squamous carcinoma has the same disadvantages as in the head and neck. Surgical resection of recurrent carcinoma is not usually possible, although it may be possible to increase the lumen size using a laser. Success in improving dysphagia by laser is independent of the histology but is improved if the obstruction involves a short length of oesophagus. Although attractive, such lasers are available in only a limited number of centres. Dilatation can be helpful, particularly if this is followed by intubation with a Celestin or Mousseau–Barbin tube (Figure 9). Endoscopic intubation carries a lower morbidity and mortality (Pfleiderer et al, 1982). Allowing such tubes to remain in place for more than a year may result in disintegration of the tube with oesophageal perforation (Hussain et al, 1987) and it has been recommended that such tubes are checked, and if necessary changed, every 6 months (Celestin, 1987). Patients with tubes should avoid dry, sticky or bulky foods and take a fizzy drink after meals.

By reducing peri-tumour oedema, corticosteroids can temporarily relieve obstructive dysphagia. Since the effect is short-term, usually a few weeks, corticosteroids are useful only in patients with total dysphagia awaiting radiotherapy or surgery, or in some patients with advanced, recurrent disease whose quality of life could be significantly improved by reducing their dysphagia in the last weeks of their lives. If swallowing problems other than obstruction are present, corticosteroids may worsen the situation by increasing appetite without relieving the dysphagia. For others, however, an improved appetite and a sense of well-being are useful side-effects.

In the series by Hanks et al (1983) candidosis was present in 31% of patients on corticosteroids, peripheral oedema in 20%, a moon face in 18%, dyspepsia in 7%, psychic changes in 4% and hyperactivity in 4%. This study found a significant correlation between the use of steroids and antifungals, however the proportion of patients with candidosis was little different to that typically seen in patients with advanced cancer. Oedema is usually mild with steroids and a filling of facial features may be welcomed by some cachectic patients. Serious psychiatric problems are uncommon but it is advisable to be wary of using steroids in patients with a previous psychiatric history. Hyperactivity, with restless legs and insomnia, can occur and may be related to the 1–3 h plasma half-life of steroids rather than to their much longer biological effect. Consequently it may be better to avoid prescribing steroids late in the day. Dyspepsia is usually mild, although up to 5% of patients with advanced cancer on steroids can develop complicated ulcer disease (Schell, 1972). A typical regimen for relieving obstructive dysphagia would be 16 mg

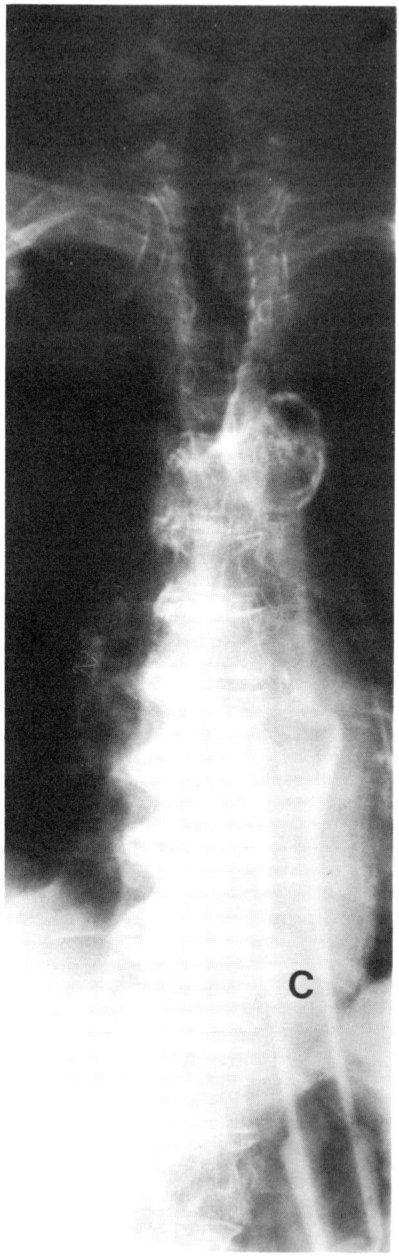

Figure 9. Celestin tube (C) inserted because of an obstructing carcinoma of lower third of oesophagus.

dexamethasone daily, increasing if necessary to 24 mg, but thereafter reducing the dose over 10 days to the lowest dose that allows swallowing. Betamethasone in the same doses is easily dissolved in water and is cheaper than soluble prednisolone. Prednisolone has the disadvantage of being a weaker corticosteroid and the starting dose of 110 mg (equivalent to 16 mg dexamethasone or betamethasone) would result in too many tablets for a dysphagic patient.

Non-oral feeding

Patients will reject a particular food consistency if they find it takes too long to swallow. If the combined oral and pharyngeal transit time is greater than 10 s with all food consistencies, patients are likely to become undernourished (Logemann, 1983). An alternative feeding route should then be considered to supplement or replace the oral route. Deciding on an appropriate route can be difficult, but some of the indications and contraindications for the different routes are shown in Table 7.

Intravenous hyperalimentation is sometimes used pre-operatively or during chemotherapy. Total parenteral nutrition requires close biochemical monitoring in hospital, but even with permanent indwelling catheters for patients at home there are practical problems of sterility in caring for the intravenous line. Other contraindications to this route include rapid deterioration, and the presence of sepsis, which is often present in head and neck cancer.

The simplest route is via a nasogastric tube. Standard tubes are inserted with some difficulty, are cosmetically unpleasant and become uncomfortable after a few days. Some patients have been taught to insert a short feeding tube for each meal (Donaldson et al, 1968), but incorrect insertion with laryngeal placement is a risk, particularly if laryngeal sensation is reduced. Soft, fine-bore, self-lubricating tubes (e.g. Clinifeed) are better tolerated. A wire introducer is needed to allow easy passage but tracheal insertion should be excluded by a chest radiograph. If correctly placed the tube tip should be seen below the diaphragm. If a radiograph is impractical a less satisfactory check can be made by injecting 20–30 ml of air into the tube and listening for bubbling sounds over the stomach with a stethoscope. Because of the risk of tracheal insertion patients should not try to insert fine-bore tubes by themselves. This is a disadvantage of fine-bore tubes since if the tube becomes dislodged the patient will have to attend a local hospital to have the tube re-positioned. In addition, displacement may be incomplete with consequent pharyngeal placement and aspiration (Boscoe and Rosin, 1984). A satisfactory solution is to insert a fine-bore or standard tube through a percutaneous cervical pharyngostomy (Meehan et al, 1984). The access is through the skin into one or other pyriform fossa and is usually performed under a short general anaesthetic, although it can be done under a local anaesthetic. Long-term placement is usually without problems, reinsertion is straightforward and unlikely to result in tracheal insertion, and the presence of the tube can be hidden by a scarf or high collar if the patient wishes.

Table 7. Indications for choosing a non-oral feeding route.

	Parenteral route	Enteral route		
		Nasogastric	Pharyngostomy/ oesophagostomy	Gastrostomy/ jejunostomy
Indications				
Oral + pharyngeal transit time > 10 s Failure to modify swallowing technique During treatment to improve muscle control Nutritional support for surgery or chemotherapy	Complete pharyngeal or oesophageal obstruction Anatomical or functional bowel loss	Short-term use (< 1 week)	Cosmetic appearance Long-term use (> 1 week)	
Contraindications				
Rapid deterioration Dysphagia due to exhaustion, debility or weakness caused by malignancy Psychological need of staff or family to provide active treatment	Presence of sepsis Limited or no access to biochemical monitoring Long-term use (> 1 month) Poor home circumstances	Abnormal nasal cavities Nasal tumour Repeated displacement	Pharyngeal or oesophageal obstruction Recently irradiated neck Superior vena caval obstruction	Jejunostomy—risk of diarrhoea, poor anaesthetic risk

A pharyngostomy is simpler than oesophagostomy, gastrostomy or jejunostomy, but these other procedures may have to be considered in obstructions below the mid-pharynx. A tube oesophagostomy (Tucker et al, 1985) is a little more complicated to fashion than a pharyngostomy, but has the advantage that tube replacement by the patient is entirely without risk of tracheal insertion. A gastrostomy can cause local skin irritation and a jejunostomy may cause diarrhoea: it is unusual for either to be considered in patients with recurrent or advanced disease.

Most tube-fed patients take intermittent feeds of high calorie liquids and there is usually little problem if this is to supplement oral feeding. In patients who depend entirely on tube feeding, the high volume of intermittent feeds can cause reflux with aspiration, together with nausea, hiccups and epigastric discomfort due to gastric distension. If the volume is reduced the high osmolality may cause hypotension and diarrhoea and there may be insufficient water to prevent dehydration. It is therefore better to start with frequent, low volume feeds and gradually build this up to larger volume feeds every 4–6 h. If diarrhoea continues to be a problem, slow or continuous administration by gravity or via a pump may help. It is also worth remembering that even with total dysphagia, patients may still enjoy tasting drinks and may find chewing food is satisfying.

Tube feeding via a pharyngostomy or oesophagostomy can provide adequate nutrition, particularly when it is supplementing the oral route, and can do so long-term with few problems.

Modifying the swallowing technique

The second factor that will affect a patient's choice of food consistency is the presence and extent of aspiration. If more than 10% of any food consistency is aspirated, patients are likely to stop eating (Logemann, 1983). Patients with severe sensory loss of the pharynx and trachea will continue to eat despite aspiration, and the extent of this aspiration can only be assessed by radiographic examination. Aspiration will either be the result of a failure in the reflexes that protect the airway, or due to excessive amounts of food or liquid in the upper pharynx due to more distal obstructions as shown in Figure 5. If there is no aspiration, or the amount aspirated is less than 10%, it may be possible to modify the swallowing technique to improve swallowing and reduce or prevent aspiration if this is occurring (Logemann, 1983; Logemann, 1985).

Swallowing may be helped by various techniques as shown in Table 8. The value of colleagues experienced in the treatment of swallowing disorders is demonstrated by the example of patients aspirating due to poor laryngeal closure. A supraglottic swallow (Table 8) is helpful and involves tilting the head back during swallowing to allow gravity to assist in moving the bolus into the oropharynx. In contrast, hemilaryngectomees may do better with the head forward during swallowing since this widens the vallecula and lessens the likelihood of aspiration. If the epiglottis has been removed, however, this technique will worsen aspiration. In addition, patients with poor laryngeal closure do better with thicker foods, but if pharyngeal

Table 8. A guide to modifying the swallowing process.

Abnormality	Action
Preparatory and oral swallowing phases	
Poor buccal control	Hand pressure on affected cheek/ place food on affected side/ tilt head to unaffected side
Abnormal mandibular movement	Hand pressure to steady mandible/ teach patient to chew bolus against hard palate/ prosthesis to correct occlusive alignment
Tongue:	
• partial glossectomy	Use liquids or soft foods/ if swallowing reflex intact—tilt head back during swallow/ syringes or glossectomy spoons (e.g. Figure 10) help carry food to the oropharynx
• reduced tongue movement	Increase tongue–bolus contact: palatal prosthesis/ if swallowing reflex intact—tilt head forward until ready to swallow then back on swallowing
• poor co-ordination	Decrease tongue–bolus contact: hold bolus against roof of mouth and swallow immediately
Reduced oral sensation	Position food in most sensitive areas/ use spices, cold foods or tastes that increase localization
Pharyngeal phase	
Delayed or absent swallowing reflex	Take small bolus and tilt head forward during swallow (opens vallecula and allows bolus more time to stimulate reflex)/ stimulate reflex with cold laryngeal mirror Consider: non-oral feeding with a programme to increase sensitivity of faucial arches by cold stimulation and increasing amounts and thickness of food
Pharynx:	
• reduced peristalsis	Follow each swallow with a liquid or dry swallow Consider: restricting consistency to liquids and thin pastes
• unilateral paralysis	Turn head to affected side (closes pyriform fossa)/ tilt head to unaffected side (directs food to normal side)
Reduced laryngeal elevation or reduced laryngeal closure	Supraglottic swallow: hold breath/ place food in mouth/ tilt head back and swallow/ cough

peristalsis is poor patients will prefer thinner foods. Hence Table 8 can only be a guide and the help of an experienced speech therapist is essential, often also with help from dental and radiologist colleagues.

Improving muscle control

If modifying the swallowing process has been unsuccessful, or if the amount of swallowed material aspirated is greater than 10%, then it may be possible to reduce dysphagia and aspiration by improving muscle control. Motor exercises can be performed to improve buccal tension, improve control of the tongue or mandible, or increase laryngeal closure. These exercises can be done in conjunction with techniques to modify swallowing and should be carried out under the advice of a speech therapist. If may be necessary for non-oral feeding to be used while these exercises are completed but those patients whose dysphagia or aspiration remains will need to continue with non-oral feeding.

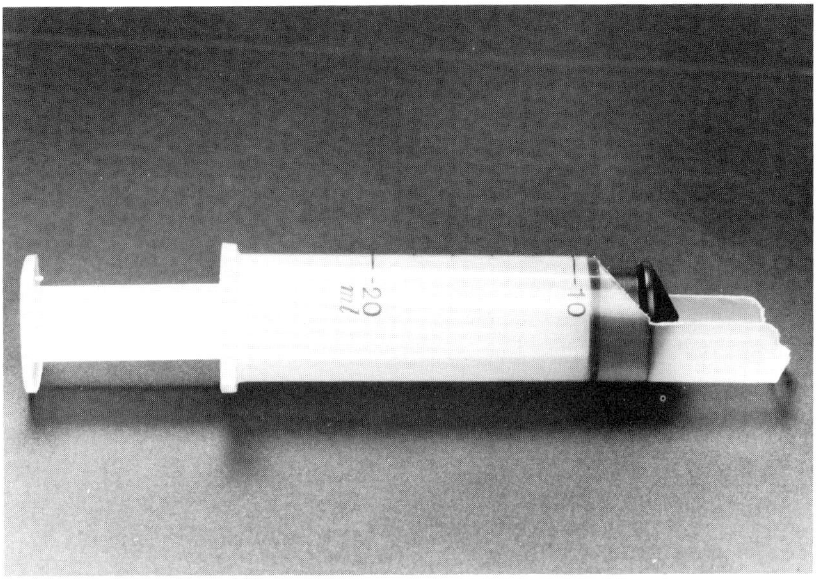

Figure 10. Glossectomy spoons help transport food past the resected tongue to a position where the swallowing reflex can be stimulated. This glossectomy feeding spoon has been made from a 20 ml plastic syringe. (Made from instructions in Fleming and Weaver, 1983.)

CONCLUSION

The complex nature of the swallowing process means there are numerous causes of its disruption. Some causes such as *Candida*, are easily diagnosed and treated. In contrast there are many causes of painful swallowing which must be differentiated, although the treatment may be straightforward. Other problems such as reduced tongue mobility will be clear to the examining clinician, but treatment may be difficult. The clinician should therefore have an understanding of normal swallowing, the effects of tumour spread such as perineural extension, and the effects on swallowing of drugs, infections, surgery, radiotherapy and chemotherapy. The clinician will then be able to make accurate diagnoses and suggest treatment, but should also be prepared to ask advice and help from nursing, speech therapy, ENT and dental colleagues.

Successful treatment of dysphagia, together with appropriate and adequate explanation to the patient, will do much to alleviate the fears of the dysphagic patient with cancer.

Acknowledgements

I am indebted to Miss Wendy Lendrem (Speech Therapist, Sanderson Centre, Newcastle-upon-Tyne), Dr Helen Lucraft (Consultant Radiotherapist, Regional Radiotherapy Centre, Newcastle-upon-Tyne), Dr Kathryn Mannix (Registrar in Palliative Care, St Oswald's

Hospice, Newcastle-upon-Tyne) and Mr Rob Ruckley (ENT Senior Registrar, Middlesbrough) for their helpful comments on the final draft of my manuscript and to Dr Simpson (Consultant Radiologist, Newcastle General Hospital, Newcastle-upon-Tyne) for his kind permission to use the X-rays illustrated, and to Yvonne Proudlock for so rapidly and skilfully mastering wordprocessing.

REFERENCES

Aird DW, Bihari J & Smith C (1983) Clinical problems in the continuing care of head and neck cancer patients. *Ear, Nose and Throat Journal* **62:** 10–30.

Ardran GM & Kemp F (1951) The mechanism of swallowing. *Proceedings of the Royal Society of Medicine* **44:** 1038–1040.

Billings JA (1985) Comfort measures for the terminally ill: is dehydration painful? *Journal of the American Geriatrics Society* **33**(11): 808–810.

Boscoe MJ & Rosin MD (1984) Fine bore enteral feeding and pulmonary aspiration. *British Medical Journal* **289:** 1421–1422.

Burnie JP, Odds FC, Lee W et al (1985a) Outbreak of systemic *Candida albicans* in intensive care unit caused by cross infection. *British Medical Journal* **290:** 746–748.

Burnie JP, Lee W, Williams JD et al (1985b) Control of an outbreak of systemic *Candida albicans*. *British Medical Journal* **291:** 1092–1093.

Carter RL, Pittman MR & Tanner NSB (1982) Pain and dysphagia in patients with squamous carcinomas of the head and neck: the role of perineural spread. *Journal of the Royal Society of Medicine* **75:** 598–606.

Celestin LR (1987) Dangers from dissolution of latex in Celestin endo-oesophageal tube. *British Medical Journal* **294:** 899.

Cohen S & Harris LD (1972) The lower esophageal sphincter. *Gastroenterology* **63**(6): 1066–1073.

Conley JJ (1960) Swallowing dysfunctions associated with radical surgery of the head and neck. *AMA Archives of Surgery* **80:** 602–612.

Dellow PG (1976) The general physiological background of chewing and swallowing. In Sessle BJ & Hannam AG (eds) *Mastication and Swallowing*, pp 6–21. Toronto: University of Toronto Press.

Dodds WJ (1976) Instrumentation and methods for intraluminal esophageal manometry. *Archives of Internal Medicine* **136**(5): 515–523.

Donaldson RC, Skelly M & Paletta FX (1968) Total glossectomy for cancer. *American Journal of Surgery* **116:** 589–590.

Duranceau A, Jamieson G, Hurwitz AL et al (1976) Alteration in esophageal motility after laryngectomy. *American Journal of Surgery* **131:** 30–35.

Editorial (1986) Terminal hydration. *Lancet* **i:** 306.

Finlay IG (1986) Oral symptoms and candida in the terminally ill. *British Medical Journal* **292:** 592–593.

Fleming SM & Weaver AW (1983) Glossectomy feeding device readily adapted from a plastic syringe. *Archives of Physical Medicine and Rehabilitation* **64:** 183–185.

Gannong WF (1977) Gastrointestinal motility and secretion. In *Review of Medical Physiology* 8th edn, pp 360–383. Los Altos: Lange Medical.

Gilmour AG & Chustecki AM (1984) Identifying oral fungal infections. *MIMS Magazine*. 1 September: 32–33.

Goldberg LJ (1976) Motorneurone mechanisms: reflex controls. In Sessle BJ & Hannam AG (eds) *Mastication and Swallowing*, pp 47–59. Toronto: University of Toronto Press.

Hanks GW, Trueman T & Twycross RG (1983) Corticosteroids in terminal cancer—a prospective analysis of current practice. *Postgraduate Medical Journal* **59:** 702–706.

Harrison DFN, Thompson AE & Buchanan G (1981) Radical resection for cancer of the hypopharynx and cervical oesophagus with repair by stomach transposition. *British Journal of Surgery* **68:** 781–783.

Hay RJ (1985) Ketoconazole: a reappraisal. *British Medical Journal* **290:** 260–261.

Hussain SA, Hughes R & Gross E (1987) Dangers from dissolution of latex in Celestin endo-oesophageal tube. *British Medical Journal* **294:** 412–413.

Kim JH, Chu F, Lakshmi V & Houde R (1985) A clinical study of benzydamine for the

treatment of radiotherapy-induced mucositis of the oropharynx. *International Journal of Tissue Reaction* **7**(3): 215–218.
Lewis JH, Zimmerman HJ, Benson GD et al (1984) Hepatic injury associated with ketoconazole therapy—analysis of 33 cases. *Gastroenterology* **86:** 503–513.
Lockhart PB & Sonis ST (1979) Relationship of oral complications to peripheral blood leukocyte and platelet counts in patients receiving cancer chemotherapy. *Oral Surgery* **48**(1): 21–28.
Logemann JA (1983) In *Evaluation and Treatment of Swallowing Disorders*. San Diego: College Hill Press.
Logemann JA (1985) Aspiration in head and neck surgical patients. *Annals of Otology, Rhinology and Laryngology* **94:** 373–376.
Logemann JA & Bytell DE (1979) Swallowing disorders in three types of head and neck surgical patients. *Cancer* **44**(3): 1095–1105.
Mantell BS (1982) Radiotherapy for dysphagia due to gastric carcinoma. *British Journal of Surgery* **69:** 69–70.
Meehan SE, Wood RAB & Cuschieri A (1984) Percutaneous cervical pharyngostomy: a comfortable and convenient alternative to protracted nasogastric intubation. *American Journal of Surgery* **148:** 325–330.
Nicolopoulos N, Mantidis A, Stathopoulos E et al (1985) Prophylactic administration for radiation oesophagitis. *Radiotherapy and Oncology* **3:** 23–25.
Ott DJ, Gelfand DW, Wu WC & Chen YM (1986) Radiological evaluation of dysphagia. *Journal of the American Medical Association* **256**(19): 2718–2721.
Pfleiderer AG, Goodall P & Holmes GKT (1982) The consequences and effectiveness of intubation in the palliation of dysphagia due to benign and malignant strictures affecting the oesophagus. *British Journal of Surgery* **69:** 356–358.
Pittam MR (1982) Does unsuccessful salvage surgery modify the terminal course of patients with squamous carcinomas of the head and neck? *Clinical Oncology* **8:** 195–200.
Regnard CFB & Davies A (1986) Pain. In *A Guide to Symptom Relief in Advanced Cancer*, 2nd edn, pp 5–18. Manchester: Haigh and Hochland.
Ritchie JR, Brown JR, Guerra LR & Mason G (1985) Dental care for the irradiated cancer patient. *Quintessence International* **12:** 837–842.
Robertson MS & Hornibrook J (1982) The presenting symptoms of head and neck cancer. *New Zealand Medical Journal* **95**(708): 337–341.
Rogers AI, Abrams KS, Presley D et al (1980) Can emotional stress induce esophageal spasm in man? *Gastroenterology* **78**(5.2): 1246.
Rowland CG & Pagliero KM (1985) Intracavitary irradiation of carcinoma of oesophagus and cardia. *Lancet* **ii:** 981–983.
Schell HW (1972) Adrenal corticosteroid therapy in far-advanced cancer. *Geriatrics* **27:** 131–141.
Sessle BJ (1976) How are mastication and swallowing programmed and regulated? In Sessle BJ & Hannam AG (eds) *Mastication and Swallowing*, pp 161–171. Toronto: University of Toronto Press.
Silverman S, Luangjarmekorn L & Greenspan D (1984) Occurrence of oral candida in irradiated head and neck cancer patients. *Journal of Oral Medicine* **39**(4): 194–196.
Sonis ST, Sonis AL & Lieberman A (1978) Oral complications in patients receiving treatment for malignancies other than of the head and neck. *Journal of the American Dental Association* **97:** 468–472.
Storey AT (1976) Interactions of alimentary and upper respiratory tract reflexes. In Sessle BJ & Hannam AG (eds) *Mastication and Swallowing*, pp 22–36. Toronto: University of Toronto Press.
Trier JS & Bjorkman DJ (1984) Esophageal, gastric and intestinal candidiasis. *American Journal of Medicine* **77**(4D): 39–43.
Tucker HM, Broniatowski M & Chase S (1985) Tube esophagostomy. *Archives of Otolaryngology* **111:** 187–189.
Twycross RG & Lack SA (1986) Dysphagia. In *Control of Alimentary Symptoms in Far Advanced Cancer*, pp 66–88. Edinburgh: Churchill Livingstone.
Veis SL & Logemann JA (1985) Swallowing disorders in persons with cerebrovascular accident. *Archives of Physical Medicine and Rehabilitation* **66:** 372–375.
Weaver AW & Fleming SM (1978) Partial laryngectomy: analysis of associated swallowing disorders. *American Journal of Surgery* **136:** 486–489.

6

Medical management of intestinal obstruction

MARY BAINES

Intestinal obstruction is caused by an occlusion to the lumen or a lack of normal propulsion which prevent or delay intestinal contents from passing distally.

Malignant obstruction can occur at any site in the gastro-intestinal tract but there are three common clinical situations:

1. Oesophageal obstruction, usually due to an oesophageal or bronchial carcinoma.
2. Gastro-duodenal obstruction, usually due to a gastric or pancreatic carcinoma.
3. Small and/or large intestinal obstruction.

This chapter is concerned solely with the third and deals with the management of intestinal obstruction.

While surgery must remain the primary treatment for malignant obstruction, it is now recognized that there is a group of patients with advanced disease or poor general condition who are unfit for surgery and require medical management. In this chapter the indications for surgery will be examined, the use of nasogastric suction and intravenous fluids evaluated and the place of drugs for symptom control described.

INCIDENCE

Intestinal obstruction is an important and common complication of malignant disease. Of 4583 patients in the Large Bowel Cancer Project 713 (16%) were obstructed and these had a significantly poorer prognosis than the remainder (Phillips et al, 1985). In 518 patients with ovarian cancer the incidence of obstruction was 127 (25%) (Tunca et al, 1981). In a survey of 1350 patients with advanced malignant disease referred to St Christopher's Hospice it was found that 40 (3%) had intestinal obstruction. The incidence was 10% in those with primary cancers of the large intestine (Baines et al, 1985).

PHYSIOLOGY

As primary tumours of the large intestine (and rarely of the small intestine) enlarge in size they may cause occlusion of the lumen. The likelihood of obstruction depends on the site, 49% of tumours at the splenic flexure obstruct, but only 6% of those in the rectum or recto-sigmoid junction (Phillips et al, 1985).

The obstruction caused by other primary tumours involving bowel, or by recurrent colorectal cancer is probably far more complex. Intraluminal obstruction is less important, but there are other major factors, several of which can co-exist.

External compression from extramural masses or malignant adhesions

Omental masses and abdominal or pelvic adhesions were found at necropsy in 12 out of 18 patients with intestinal obstruction (Table 1) (Baines et al, 1985). These caused external compression of the bowel but did not penetrate into the lumen.

The radiological diagnosis of metastatic disease causing obstruction in gynaecological malignancy is based on finding an extramucosal mass or masses producing deformity or kinking of loops of bowel (Yuhasz et al, 1985).

Multiple sites of obstruction

In Hospice patients who have died with intestinal obstruction from advanced malignant disease, it is usual to find multiple sites of obstruction. These were present in 14 out of 18 autopsies. In 10 cases the small intestine was involved in several places, in 4 cases the small and large intestine (Table 1).

Table 1. Distribution of abdominal and pelvic tumour at necropsy in 18 patients with intestinal obstruction.

Site of primary tumour	Main sites of tumour found at necropsy	Level(s) of intestinal obstruction: Multiple SI	Multiple SI and LI	Single SI	Single LI
Ovary(3) Stomach(1)	Omentum(4)	2	2	0	0
Ovary(2) Colon(2) Rectum(2) Stomach(1) Endometrium(1)	Abdominal and/or pelvic adhesions(8)	6	2	0	0
Ovary(3) Rectum(1)	Pelvis(4)	1	0	1	2
Colon(2)	Other(2)	1	0	1	0

Numbers in parentheses = number of patients.
SI = small intestine.
LI = large intestine.

Infiltration of intestinal muscle

Lateral spread of tumour within the muscle coats is sometimes found causing an 'intestinal *linitis plastica*'. This can transform the bowel into a rigid malfunctioning tube.

Neurogenic obstruction

Pseudo-obstruction is a condition which presents the signs and symptoms of bowel obstruction without a mechanical block. There are many causes of this condition, but it has been described with malignant infiltration of the autonomic nerves of the coeliac plexus on the posterior abdominal wall (Addison, 1983). Experience in performing coeliac axis blocks for upper abdominal pain in cancer patients confirms that the coeliac axis is sometimes infiltrated with tumour.

Obstruction of venous and lymphatic drainage

This is thought to be due to peritoneal seeding on bowel and mesentery, causing motility disorders in cases of advanced ovarian cancer (Osteen et al, 1980).

Nickell and Dockerty (1948) suggest other causes contributing to obstruction: a change in colonic flora in the proximal segment (by the production of gas); inflammatory oedema; impaction of solid faeces; fatigue of intestinal muscle above the point of stenosis; the elasticity of the intestinal wall and the amount of fibrosis present. To these must be added the constipating effect of many drugs.

Thus the physiology of malignant intestinal obstruction is often multifactorial. There may be a mechanical block from intraluminal tumour or external compression; there may be a functional component from malignant involvement of intestinal muscle or autonomic nerves; the obstruction may be at several sites; it may be precipitated by inflammatory oedema or the effect of constipating drugs.

Strangulation, or ischaemia of the bowel, is commonly found in obstruction due to hernia or adhesion, but is very rarely found in malignant intestinal obstruction. Three series reported an incidence of 4% or less (Zadeh et al, 1985; Bizer et al, 1981 and Osteen et al, 1980).

AETIOLOGY

There are many papers giving the types of primary tumours which cause intestinal obstruction. Unfortunately they are not easily comparable, some include benign causes of obstruction, some are from surgeons, others from gynaecologists. Some series deal only with small bowel obstruction, others with both small and large bowel obstruction, for these can often co-exist in patients with advanced cancer.

The surgical series contain relatively few cases of ovarian cancer, but a high incidence of patients with primary cervical cancer in whom the obstruction is usually caused by post-irradiation fibrosis. The series from Walsh and Schofield (1984) (Table 2) reviewed patients presenting with small bowel obstruction after radical treatment of malignancy. They found that 32% had obstruction due to causes other than recurrent tumour, this was predominantly in cases of carcinoma of cervix or bladder following pelvic radiotherapy. There were a few cases of benign adhesions or a second primary tumour.

Table 2. Aetiology of small bowel obstruction—surgical series.

Primary tumour	Total	Recurrent	Non-recurrent
Cervix	14	3	11
Bladder	6	3	3
Colorectal	15	13	2
Ovary	7	6	1
Lymphoma	8	8	0
Others	3	3	0

From Walsh and Schofield (1984), with permission.

Ketcham et al (1970) in a similar series reported that 26% of their patients had intestinal obstruction not caused by metastatic disease, but again 26% had primary cancer of cervix.

The series from St Christopher's Hospice was based on 40 consecutive patients (16 men, 24 women) referred to the Hospice for terminal care by their general practitioners or hospital consultants. They were aged 26–94 years (mean 59). The sites of primary tumour are shown in Table 3. They include both surgical and gynaecological malignancies, both small and large bowel obstruction. Of course, patients with a benign cause for obstruction would not be referred for Hospice care unless it was felt that their poor general condition precluded surgery.

Table 3. Sites of primary tumours in 40 patients with intestinal obstruction—St Christopher's Hospice series.

Site of primary carcinoma	Number	Male	Female
Ovary	14	0	14
Rectum	8	5	3
Colon	8	7	1
Caecum	2	1	1
Stomach	2	1	1
Endometrium	1	0	1
Prostate	1	1	0
Bladder	1	0	1
Mesothelium (peritoneum)	1	0	1
Unknown	3	1	2

One patient had 2 primary carcinomas, rectum and colon.

CLINICAL FEATURES

Malignant intestinal obstruction may present acutely with the sudden onset of colicky abdominal pain, nausea and vomiting and constipation. Physical examination will then show abdominal distension and hyperactive, high pitched bowel sounds.

However, more often the onset of obstruction is insidious, over weeks or months. Symptoms may gradually worsen and become continuous but, even without treatment, symptoms may be intermittent and the obstructive episodes resolve spontaneously. The distinction is often made between complete or partial (subacute) obstruction but this is far from easy in practice and the obstruction may clinically appear to alter from one to the other on several occasions as the illness progresses.

In the series from St Christopher's Hospice the symptomatology was as follows:

Nausea and vomiting	100%
Intestinal colic	76%
Other abdominal pain (due to distension or tumour masses)	92%
Diarrhoea	34%

Only 13% specifically mentioned constipation as a symptom.

The signs of chronic intestinal obstruction vary considerably. Abdominal distension is usually present, but will be absent in jejunal involvement. More importantly, there may be minimal distension if the small bowel is extensively infiltrated and fixed by tumour, when the abdomen will have a uniformly stiff and doughy feel (Taylor, 1985). High pitched, 'tinkling' bowel sounds may be present, but a common finding, of which patients often complain, is loud bursts of borborygmi coming intermittently. The presence of hepatomegaly, tumour masses or ascites must be noted as they will affect plans for treatment.

DIFFERENTIAL DIAGNOSIS

The differential diagnosis of intestinal obstruction in a patient previously treated for cancer is as follows:

Constipation. This is common in cancer patients, being aggravated by inactivity, a diet low in roughage and by analgesic and other drugs.

Benign causes. These include adhesions, post-irradiation bowel damage, inflammatory bowel disease and hernia. In Walsh and Schofield's series (1984) no less than 15 of their 53 patients with small bowel obstruction had benign causes.

Malignant causes. There may be recurrence of the previous tumour or a new primary, with a better prognosis, may be the cause of obstruction.

Constipation

This should be suspected as the cause of obstruction if there is a history of increasingly hard faeces, infrequent defaecation and the use of constipating drugs, such as morphine, without a concomitant laxative.

Physical examination usually shows a loaded rectum and faecal masses palpable abdominally but occasionally, with a high impaction, the rectum is empty. It may be difficult to distinguish between malignant and faecal masses felt abdominally. Investigations are rarely needed for diagnosis, but plain abdominal X-rays show faecal masses, occasionally leading to distension and fluid levels.

The treatment of faecal impaction is firstly with local measures, suppositories and enemas. These should be followed with laxatives, the combination of a faecal softener and a stimulant, such as lactulose and senna being found the most effective.

It must be remembered that a few cases, thought to be severe constipation, are due to a progressive subacute obstruction.

Benign and malignant obstruction

It is often difficult to distinguish between these and the diagnosis is frequently not made until laparotomy. However, there are some indicators:

Primary tumours. Certain tumours are known to involve the bowel causing obstruction, others do so very rarely. Yuhasz et al (1985) found that small bowel complications in patients with ovarian cancers were invariably due to metastatic disease, while in cervical cancer small bowel disease was usually due to radiation damage.

Clinical history. Unless there is a very long history suggestive of a benign cause, the symptoms do not help in diagnosis. However, the results of previous abdominal surgery will often point to the cause of obstruction.

Physical examination. This may show abdominal tumour masses or the doughy abdomen of disseminated disease. Sigmoidoscopy as well as rectal examination may be necessary.

Straight abdominal X-rays. These confirm obstruction but are often unhelpful in elucidating the cause.

Barium studies. A small bowel enema can usually distinguish between obstruction from metastases, radiation bowel damage and adhesions, (Yuhasz et al, 1985). The slow passage of barium through undilated bowel with no demonstrable point of obstruction points to a motility disorder as found in ovarian cancer (Osteen et al, 1980). A barium enema is used to delineate large bowel obstruction.

In practice, there is no value in subjecting the patient to abdominal X-rays or barium studies if his poor general condition precludes surgical intervention.

MANAGEMENT

Surgery

Every cancer patient who develops intestinal obstruction must be considered for surgery. This includes those referred to a hospice for terminal care since even if the obstruction is due to recurrent cancer there are individuals who will enjoy a long and symptom-free period following palliative surgery.

Indications for surgery

1. The possibility of a single, remediable block, either malignant or benign.
2. Good general condition.
3. Absence of large abdominal tumour masses.
4. Marked abdominal distension. This has been described by Taylor (1985). They found that the feasibility of palliative surgery can be predicted from a careful physical examination and erect abdominal X-rays. If the degree of distension is modest and the abdomen has a stiff, doughy feel, then the erect film usually shows very small fluid levels dispersed over the whole abdomen. This is due to extensive infiltration and fixation of the small bowel and palliation is unlikely to be possible. If, however, the upper abdomen is very distended, not uniformly doughy, and two or more loops of bowel can be seen on the erect X-ray, surgery is usually feasible.
5. The patient's wish for surgery.

Contraindications to surgery

These are poor general condition, the presence of multiple sites of obstruction or the patient's refusal.

In the St Christopher's Hospice series of 40 patients, only two were considered suitable for surgery. The remaining 38 were managed medically for the following reasons:

Previous laparotomy for obstruction—no procedure possible	10
Previous surgical opinion	12
Extensive intra-abdominal disease	9
Too old or too ill	5
Surgery refused	2

No patient was referred for surgery simply to prevent a distressing death from obstruction. The correct use of drugs has made this unnecessary and probably influenced surgical policy in surrounding general hospitals.

Case history. Mrs R E (aged 63) had been treated by repeated diathermy for a transitional cell carcinoma of the bladder for 11 years, when a massive pelvic recurrence was found. Total cystectomy with a transverse colon conduit was performed, followed by pelvic irradiation. Three months later she developed complete large bowel obstruction due to recurrent pelvic tumour, causing constipation, colic and vomiting. In addition to her malignancy, Mrs R E had an above-knee amputation of her right leg, following a war injury, and a left hemiplegia. The possibility of a colostomy was discussed with the patient, but she declined it, requesting only palliative treatment. After transfer to St Christopher's Hospice she was started on a continuous subcutaneous infusion of diamorphine and haloperidol, using the syringe driver. Until her death 16 days later, the pain and vomiting were controlled by an increase in the analgesia to diamorphine 40 mg/24 hours, and a change to methotrimeprazine 50–100 mg/24 hours, as the anti-emetic.

Other series, with fewer ill patients, show a far higher incidence of surgical palliation of intestinal obstruction. In four series the operative rate was between 71% and 87%.

Appropriate surgical procedures vary greatly, sometimes resection of tumour is possible, more often a bypass procedure is done or a colostomy or ileostomy formed.

The results of surgical palliation of malignant obstruction are shown in Table 4. Operative mortality is considerable and survival is usually measured in months. In the St Christopher's Hospice series the mean survival of 11 patients after palliative surgery was 7 months, but four continued to have obstructive symptoms. Ketcham et al (1970) reported a re-obstruction rate of 33%.

In practice, therefore, the decision to proceed to surgery requires careful discussion, involving medical and nursing staff, the patient and family. There will be many patients who are old or very ill who request only symptomatic treatment. Others, particularly the young, will want every chance of prolongation of life, especially if there is effective chemotherapy available following surgery.

Case history. Mrs A C (aged 35). This patient was investigated for infertility, an ovarian cyst was found but not biopsied. She was treated with clomiphene and conceived. During pregnancy she complained of pain and a pelvic mass was diagnosed. After the birth at 34 weeks a laparotomy was performed which showed stage four ovarian cancer. She was treated with cisplatin (cisplatinum) with a partial response. Five months after laparotomy she developed obstructive symptoms. Abdominal X-rays indicated a single

Table 4. Results of palliative surgical treatment for malignant intestinal obstruction.

Author	Number of patients	Primary tumours	Operative mortality (%)	Faecal fistulae (%)	Median survival (months)
Aranha et al	73	Various	31	10	6 (mean)
Osteen et al	32	Various	—	—	3
Piver et al	60	Ovary	32	7	2.5
Tunca et al	127	Ovary	14	—	7 (mean)
Walsh and Schofield	36	Various	19	—	11

sigmoid obstruction and this was confirmed at laparotomy when a colostomy was performed. She received further chemotherapy, but with no response and she died at home, without re-obstructing, 3 months later.

Intravenous fluids and nasogastric suction

This is the conventional primary treatment for any patient admitted to hospital suffering with symptoms and signs of obstruction. The value of this treatment to decompress the bowel and correct fluid and electrolyte imbalance before surgery is proven, but its use as the sole means of treating malignant obstruction is questionable. A review of the literature is shown in Table 5.

Table 5. Response of obstructed patients to intravenous fluids and nasogastric suction.

Author	Number of patients	Sustained response (%)	Comment
Aranha et al	73	1	'Tube decompression rarely effective.'
Bizer et al	35	14	'Consider early surgery in malignant disease.'
Ketcham et al	86		'Conservative management seldom indicated.'
Osteen et al	66	14	21 (32%) patients had benign obstruction
Piver et al	60		'No relief by tube decompression.'
Walsh and Schofield	36		'A policy of operation after adequate rehydration.'

It is perhaps surprising that the percentage reported response to conservative treatment is so low. It is well recognized and was noted in the St Christopher's Hospice series that early obstructive symptoms can be intermittent. It is probable that some patients whose symptoms resolved with intravenous fluids and nasogastric suction would have improved spontaneously or with symptomatic treatment using appropriate medication.

The place of prolonged conservative treatment in a patient with unresolved malignant obstruction is controversial. Such treatment involves hospitalization, immobility and discomfort. It is a barrier between patient and family at a time when they most need each other's closeness and support. The statement 'Prolonged conservative management using nasogastric suction and intravenous fluids only adds to the discomfort of an already terminally ill patient' (Aranha et al, 1981) is undoubtedly true. Hospice policy is to treat these patients symptomatically, with appropriate drugs. They are then free to eat and drink as they wish, move about the ward with ease or be cared for at home.

Symptomatic treatment

If surgery is considered inappropriate and long-term conservative management adds to patient distress, a new approach is needed to the management of patients with malignant intestinal obstruction. At St Christopher's Hospice these patients have been treated symptomatically since 1967 and the drug regimens described have gradually evolved (Baines, 1984).

Before consideration of the effective drugs, it is important to be familiar with the various routes of administration:

1. Oral. If vomiting is absent or infrequent.
2. Sublingual. Only a few drugs available.
3. Rectal. Useful in the home, may be impossible in pelvic malignancies, a limited number of drugs are made in suppository form.
4. Intramuscular. Can be used occasionally, but repeated injections, in the emaciated patient, are painful and difficult.
5. Intravenous. Continuous intravenous fluids are not recommended.
6. Subcutaneous. This route is preferred if the patient is vomiting.

The Graseby Medical portable syringe driver allows the continuous infusion of parenteral medication subcutaneously. Many drugs can be given by this route and it is ideal for use in the home as the drugs can be loaded every 24 hours by the visiting nurse (Oliver, 1985a).

The symptoms of obstruction have been described previously and the management of each will be presented separately.

Intestinal colic

This was reported in 76% of patients.

Treatment options:

1. Discontinue stimulant laxatives e.g. bisacodyl and senna.
2. Discontinue metoclopramide and domperidone, these may increase peristalsis in the small intestine.
3. Analgesics such as codeine, morphine or diamorphine are sometimes effective alone.
4. Usually the addition of an antispasmodic is required.
5. If no vomiting, try loperamide 2–4 mg four times daily or sublingual hyoscine 0.3–0.6 mg as required for occasional colic.
6. If vomiting is a problem, drugs should be given by continuous subcutaneous infusion. Hyoscine 0.8 mg/24 hours, increasing slowly to 2 mg/24 hours is usually effective. Atropine can be substituted if hyoscine causes unacceptable sedation.
7. A coeliac axis block, using bupivacaine or alcohol gave relief in three out of five patients.

With these treatments 31% continued to have mild colic, the remainder were pain free.

Case history. Mr N M (aged 40) developed symptoms of intestinal obstruction two and a half years after an abdomino-perineal resection for carcinoma of the rectum. Laparotomy showed malignant adhesions in the pelvis, involving the terminal ileum, and an ileocolic anastomosis was performed. After 3 months he obstructed again and was treated conservatively during repeated hospital admission over the next 6 months. On admission to St Christopher's Hospice he complained of episodes of severe colic associated with vomiting. The colic was partially relieved by sublingual hyoscine 0.6 mg as necessary. A coeliac plexus block reduced the severity of the colic, but he continued to require hyoscine on occasions. A syringe driver with hyoscine 0.8–1.6 mg/24 hours was started as his condition deteriorated to maintain control of increasing colic. Post mortem examination showed dilated bowel obstruction by malignant adhesions in the right iliac and suprapubic regions.

Other abdominal pain

This was reported in 92% of patients. It was due to abdominal distension, hepatomegaly or tumour masses.

Treatment options:

1. If there was minimal vomiting, oral morphine or diamorphine was given. They can be given in a mixture with chloroform water every 4 hours or as morphine sulphate continus (MST) every 12 hours. The dose should be increased until pain control is achieved.
2. If vomiting is a problem and suppositories are acceptable, oxycodone pectinate (Proladone) 30–60 mg every 8 hours is often effective.
3. For more severe pain associated with vomiting the subcutaneous route is preferred. Diamorphine is the strong opioid of choice because of its great solubility.
4. Coeliac axis block.

With these treatments, 89% of patients became pain free, in the remainder the pain was mild.

Case history. Mrs M S (aged 58) was found to have a disseminated ovarian carcinoma at laparotomy. There were tumour deposits on the surface of the large and small bowel, partial colonic obstruction, and hepatic and omental metastases. Bilateral salpingo-oophorectomy was performed. She was thought to be too ill for chemotherapy, and was discharged home at her request. She complained of central abdominal pain and the abdomen was distended and tender. Oxycodone suppositories were started at 30 mg 6 hourly, and increased later to 60 mg 6 hourly, with prochlorperazine suppositories 6 hourly for nausea. When the vomiting worsened a syringe driver was started with methotrimeprazine and diamorphine 60–120 mg/24 hours. She remained at home, her pain well controlled, until her death 8 weeks after surgery.

Vomiting

This was present in 100% of patients, being moderate or severe in 87%. Severity depended on the level of obstruction and there was considerable nausea. The vomiting usually started by being intermittent but it could become almost continuous and faeculent.

Treatment options:

1. Prochlorperazine suppositories 25 mg 8 hourly or chlorpromazine suppositories 50–100 mg 8 hourly.
2. If suppositories are unacceptable or ineffective, the subcutaneous route is used. Haloperidol 5 mg/24 hours increasing slowly to 15 mg/24 hours is usually effective. (Parkinsonian side-effects may occur at higher doses.)
3. Cyclizine 50 mg 8 hourly rectally or 100–150 mg/24 hours subcutaneously can be added to options 1 or 2.
4. The most effective anti-emetic in obstructive vomiting has been found to be methotrimeprazine (Nozinan), 50–150 mg/24 hours given subcutaneously. However, the drug has two disadvantages: it usually causes sedation (Oliver, 1985b), and subcutaneous irritation occurs, necessitating site changes every few days.
5. Dietary advice. Patients are allowed to eat and drink as they choose, the majority favouring small and mainly fluid meals. With adequate oral fluids, thirst is rarely a problem and the occasional dry mouth is treated with local measures such as crushed ice to suck. Electrolytes are only occasionally checked, but remain remarkably normal.

With these treatments, 13% of patients stopped vomiting, 76% had mild vomiting (not more than one episode per day with little or no nausea). Many had previously received conventional conservative treatment for intestinal obstruction. All preferred the use of appropriate anti-emetics to the re-insertion of a nasogastric tube.

Case history. Mr A H (aged 37) had required a right hemicolectomy for carcinoma of the hepatic flexure of the colon. After 10 months he developed colicky abdominal pain, distension and vomiting. At laparotomy no procedure was possible as there were multiple malignant adhesions. During the next 4 months he was treated conservatively for intestinal obstruction on three occasions. Before admission to the Hospice the intravenous fluids had been discontinued and he was started on regular suppositories of oxycodone pectinate and chlorpromazine. Eight days after admission to the Hospice the vomiting recurred and became faeculent, in association with colic and generalized abdominal pain. A syringe driver was started, and the vomiting was eased with methotrimeprazine 50–150 mg/24 hours until his death 23 days later. He vomited on alternate days, but continued to enjoy eating small amounts of food. Post mortem examination showed multiple levels of obstruction, with gross dilatation of large and small bowel, due to widespread malignant adhesions.

Diarrhoea

This was present in 34% of patients, a third of these had faecal fistulae, either enterocutaneous or enterovaginal. The diarrhoea of subacute obstruction sometimes continued until death, sometimes it preceded complete obstruction.

Treatment was with conventional antidiarrhoeal drugs, loperamide and codeine. Excluding the patients with fistulae, 56% of the remainder were controlled.

Constipation

Only 13% of patients specifically mentioned this symptom. It was treated only in the few patients in whom a single colonic or rectal obstruction was suspected. Stimulant purgatives and high enemas were avoided and faecal-softening laxatives given such as magnesium hydroxide and liquid paraffin emulsion (Milpar), docusate or an arachis oil retention enema.

PROGNOSIS

The prognosis of patients with malignant obstruction, after they have received palliative surgery, has already been discussed. Many of the papers referred to also give the prognoses for patients unfit for surgery, or who received only laparotomy and biopsy. However, the time span in these cases dates from hospital admission or surgery, not from the onset of obstruction.

In the series from St Christopher's Hospice a careful attempt was made to date the first obstructive symptoms so that the natural history of intestinal obstruction, in the absence of relieving surgery, could be determined. The results are shown in Figure 1.

The mean survival was 3.7 months. Seven patients lived with intestinal obstruction for 7 months or more. The following were thought to be contributing factors:

1. Effective chemotherapy. Two patients with ovarian cancer received cisplatin.
2. Faecal fistula formation.
3. Localized rectal carcinoma.
4. Slowly growing tumours. Three young patients with disseminated colorectal cancers survived for 7–9 months.

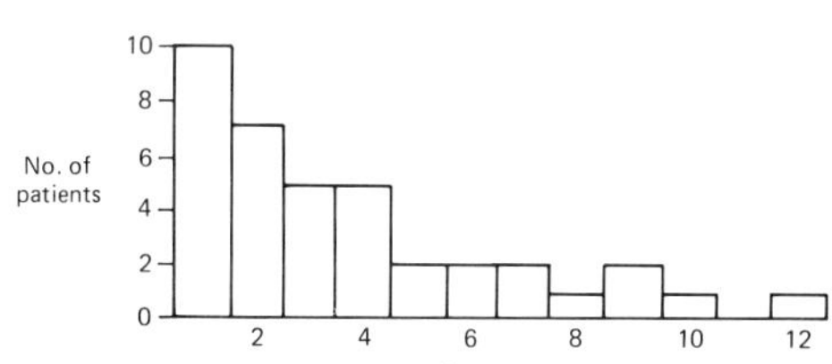

Figure 1. Survival time (months) of patients with intestinal obstruction.

The importance of effective chemotherapy has already been referred to and is confirmed in other reports. Piver et al (1982) for example found that patients who responded to postoperative chemotherapy for carcinoma of the ovary had a median survival of 10 months, whereas those with progressive disease lived only 3 months.

SUMMARY

Malignant intestinal obstruction is a common complication in patients with colorectal or ovarian cancer; it can also occur in other malignancies. Obstruction from intraluminal tumour occurs in large bowel cancer but the pathophysiology of obstruction by other primary tumours, or recurrent colorectal cancer, is probably more complex. External compression can involve multiple sites and there may be a functional component from malignant involvement of bowel muscle, autonomic nerves and lymphatic drainage.

It is important not to assume that all cases of intestinal obstruction in patients treated for cancer are due to recurrent tumour. Benign causes may occur, especially following irradiation, or a second primary tumour may develop. Severe constipation in the cancer patient, especially those receiving opiates, can mimic obstruction.

Malignant obstruction may present acutely but more often the onset is gradual and, at first, the symptoms may be intermittent. Vomiting, colic, abdominal pain and bowel disturbance all occur, but abdominal distension may be minimal if there is extensive tumour infiltration.

Surgery remains the primary treatment if the patient is well enough and if there is the possibility of a single, remediable block. Unfortunately, many cancer patients are too ill or have widespread abdominal disease. Intravenous fluids and nasogastric suction are of value prior to surgery but there is little evidence that they relieve obstruction and they add to patient distress if continued long-term.

Studies have shown that most obstructive symptoms can be relieved by appropriate drugs. Intestinal colic and other abdominal pain can be relatively easily controlled; vomiting is more difficult but it can usually be reduced to once or twice a day with little associated nausea. Patients are therefore able to move about or be cared for at home.

Although the onset of malignant obstruction means that the prognosis is short, the distressing symptoms of this condition can be adequately controlled by drugs.

Acknowledgements

I am grateful to Dr R. Carter and Dr D. Oliver for their advice. They were co-authors of the paper on the Medical Management of Intestinal Obstruction referred to in this chapter.

REFERENCES

Addison NV (1983) Pseudo-obstruction of the large bowel. *Journal of the Royal Society of Medicine* **76:** 252–255.

Aranha GV, Folk FA & Greenlee HB (1981) Surgical palliation of small bowel obstruction due to metastatic carcinoma. *American Surgeon* **47:** 99–102.

Baines MJ (1984) Control of other symptoms. In Saunders CM (ed.) *The Management of Terminal Malignant Disease*, pp 100–132. London: Edward Arnold.

Baines M, Oliver DJ & Carter RL (1985) Medical management of intestinal obstruction in patients with advanced malignant disease: a clinical and pathological study. *Lancet* **ii:** 990–993.

Bizer LS, Liebling RW, Delany HM & Gliedman ML (1981) Small bowel obstruction. *Surgery* **89**(4): 407–413.

Ketcham AS, Hoye RC, Pilch YH & Morton DL (1970) Delayed intestinal obstruction following treatment for cancer. *Cancer* **25:** 406–410.

Nickell DF & Dockerty MB (1948) The five year survival rate in cases of completely obstructing annular carcinoma of the descending colon and sigmoid. *Surgery, Gynecology and Obstetrics* **87:** 519.

Oliver DJ (1985a) The use of the syringe driver in terminal care. *British Journal of Clinical Pharmacology* **20:** 515–516.

Oliver DJ (1985b) The use of methotrimeprazine in terminal care. *British Journal of Clinical Practice* **39:** 339–340.

Osteen RT, Guyton S, Steele G & Wilson RE (1980) Malignant intestinal obstruction. *Surgery* **67:** 611–615.

Phillips RKS, Hittinger R, Fry JS & Fielding LP (1985) Malignant large bowel obstruction. *British Journal of Surgery* **72:** 296–302.

Piver MS, Barlow JJ, Lele SB & Frank A (1982) Survival after ovarian cancer induced intestinal obstruction. *Gynecologic Oncology* **13:** 44–49.

Taylor RH (1985) Laparotomy for obstruction with recurrent tumour (letter). *British Journal of Surgery* **72**(4): 327.

Tunca JC, Buchler DA & Mack EA (1981) The management of ovarian-cancer-caused bowel obstruction. *Gynecologic Oncology* **12:** 186–192.

Walsh HP & Schofield PF (1984) Is laparotomy for small bowel obstruction justified in patients with previously treated malignancy? *British Journal of Surgery* **71:** 933–935.

Yuhasz M, Laufer I, Sutton G, Herlinger H & Caroline D (1985) Radiography of the small bowel in patients with gynecologic malignancies. *American Journal of Radiology* **144:** 303–307.

Zadeh BJ, Davis JM & Canizaro PC (1985) Small bowel obstruction in the elderly. *American Surgeon* **51:** 470–473.

7

Confusion

AVERIL STEDEFORD

When a nurse or relative reports that a patient has become confused, the doctor usually feels obliged to do something about it and is often tempted to respond almost immediately with a prescription, probably for chlorpromazine. This temptation should be firmly resisted. First he should find out what the patient has been doing or saying that has led to this 'diagnosis' and he should then assess the patient for himself. A wide variety of behaviours may be described such as wandering, getting into the wrong bed, or mistaking staff for relatives, all of which suggest that the patient is not fully aware of where he is, the time of day, or the identity of those around him. He may be forgetful or uninhibited. He may be frightened or noisy and aggressive because he is hallucinating or deluded, behaving in a way that seems irrational to everyone else but is an entirely appropriate response to his world as he is perceiving it. The approach to such a patient must be on two levels.

1. A tentative diagnosis of the cause must be made so that investigations can be done if necessary and specific treatment instituted wherever possible.
2. Reaching an understanding of the patient's experience and behaviour will make management easier and more effective.

Many clinicians find confused patients bewildering and even frightening. This attitude on our part exacerbates the situation because it increases the patient's fear that what is happening to him is incomprehensible, mad, and out of control. To feel understood is important for these patients, as almost all of them are lucid for at least part of the time and are at those moments worried by the recognition that 'I am not my usual self, doctor'. Understanding is especially important when the cause of confusion is not reversible, or during the hours or days while the disturbance is being brought under control. The anxiety of staff and relatives can be reduced by explanation, allowing them to adopt a more confident and flexible attitude.

A model first used in the study of schizophrenia is helpful in understanding many of the experiences of confused patients. It postulates that there is a 'filter' which circumscribes awareness. This filter controls the entry of information from the outside world via the sense organs, from the body via pain and proprioceptive pathways, and from the unconscious. To be aware of, for example, every sound, the touch of clothes, the heart beat, and all the contents of the memory store would be totally overwhelming and it is

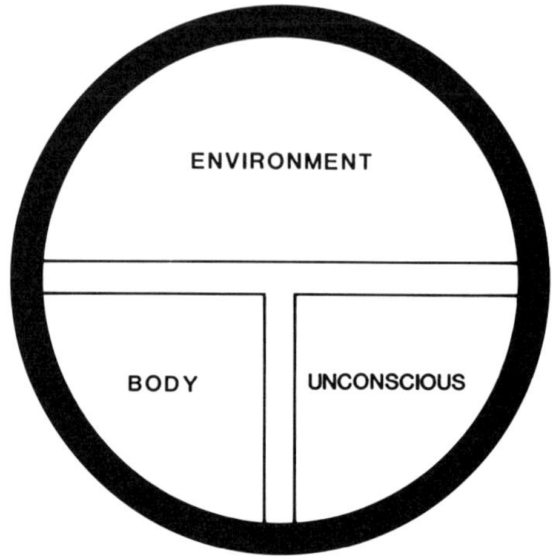

Figure 1. The filter circumscribing awareness.

essential for normal functioning that most of this is excluded. The hypothetical filter that does this is represented by the circumference of the circle in Figure 1.

The area of awareness within the circle is partitioned to indicate that people normally know from which of the three sources information is coming at any one time. The filter permits selection and allows the intensity of the experience to be varied in the same way that a radio has both tuning and volume control.

It can be seen from Figure 2 that the level of arousal is like volume control and that 'set' allows for selectivity. This concept of set is best explained by examples. A person who has been sitting by the fire-side listening to ghost stories has a fearful emotional set. In this situation the creak of the stairs or

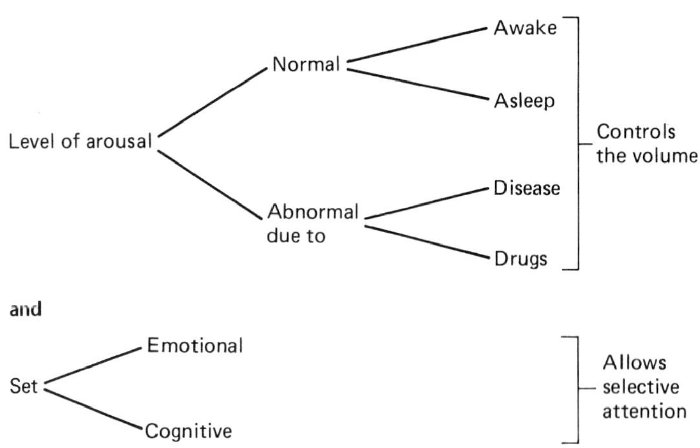

Figure 2. Factors influencing permeability of the filter.

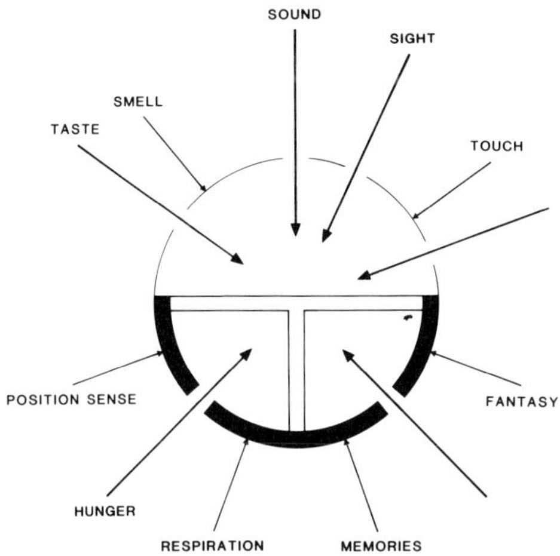

Figure 3. The normal person: awake.

the flap of the curtain in a night breeze may be startling, whereas in other circumstances it would pass almost unnoticed. A mother who knows that her baby is ill and might vomit in the night (her cognitive set) will sleep soundly through loud traffic but would waken at the baby's slightest stirring.

Figure 3 represents a normal person when awake. The filter is thin in the top half of the circle to indicate that most experience enters from the environment. Only those bodily sensations that require action, such as hunger or a full bladder, reach awareness, and the person has considerable control over what he is thinking about and remembering, although thoughts and memories irrelevant to the task in hand do intrude from time to time. This ability to control thinking is usually referred to as concentration. The partitions between the segments are intact, indicating that the person is able to separate stimuli from various sources.

Figure 4 represents the normal person when asleep. Most experience comes from the unconscious in the form of dreams, and almost all stimuli from the environment and the body are excluded. Only those stimuli which require action get through. The partitions are incomplete. A full bladder may provoke a disturbed dream before the person awakes, and anyone who has been 'on call' knows how the ring of a telephone may be woven into the story of the dream in the moments just before waking.

Figure 5 represents confusion. Impairment of consciousness, for whatever cause, decreases the permeability of the filter for environmental stimuli. Awareness of the body seems to be increased or distorted, and material that usually remains unconscious may appear as vivid memories or hallucinations. The partitions break down and the patient may be inaccurate in his perception of the source of his experience. It is understandable that he may be distressed or terrified and behave accordingly. Those around him who have no idea what his inner world is like at the moment are baffled and may feel helpless.

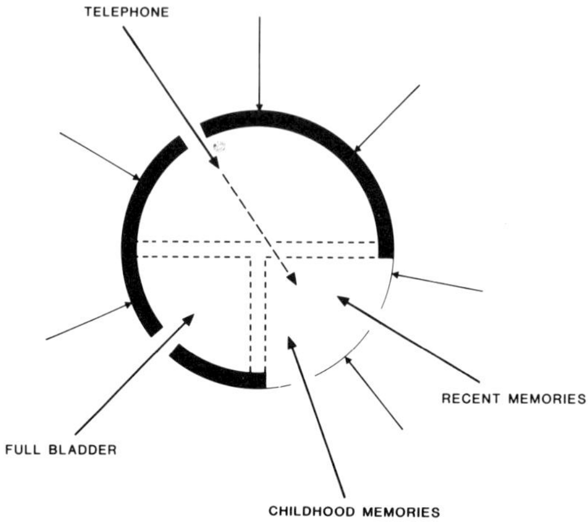

Figure 4. The normal person: asleep.

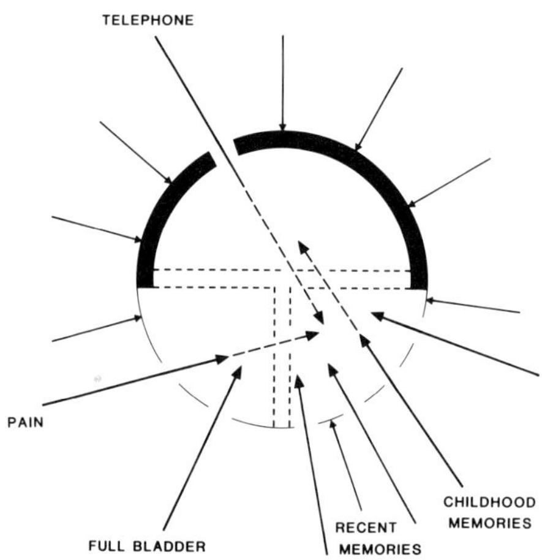

Figure 5. Confusion.

Table 1. Components of disturbed experiences.

Patient	Level of arousal	Stimulus	Set		Experience
1	Deeply asleep	High temperature	Afraid of death	⟶	Nightmare of burning to death
2	Drugged	Stranger	Guilty	⟶	Misperception of stranger as a policeman; attempts to escape
3	Drowsy	Stranger	Longing to see mother	⟶	Misperception of stranger as mother

Table 1 shows how three common experiences may come about when the factors of lowered arousal, incoming stimuli, and set are combined. Patient number 1 (who is deeply asleep, feverish, and knows that he has a condition from which he may soon die), has a nightmare that he is burning to death. From the table, the components of treatment are obvious: wake him up as fully as possible and treat his fever, which may be sufficient to calm him down. But it is not always so, and in this situation he may respond to a gentle invitation to talk about anything that is frightening him. When fear is suppressed or denied, it may sometimes find expression in this way as a recurrent nightmare. It is preferable to explore such fears with the patient there and then, if he is willing. By the next morning he may have forgotten them or be reluctant to talk about them further. Nightmares like this often cease when the underlying fear has been openly recognized.

Patients who are seriously ill often review their lives and some feel guilty about aspects of their past. If their consciousness is impaired, they may mistakenly think a stranger is someone who has come to arrest or punish them, and they may attempt to escape (patient number 2). Some of these patients may be helped by a priest or psychotherapist in whom they can confide, and who will help them to accept what has happened and perhaps attempt reconciliation or to make amends. Patients also think about good memories. They are often living in the past and expect to see relatives with whom they have been close. If such a person is drowsy, he may think that a nurse who approaches the bedside is his mother (patient number 3). The nurse then has to decide how she will respond. If she does not correct the misperception and the patient becomes lucid, he may realize his mistake and feel angry that he is being humoured. A better alternative might be to say gently 'No, I am not your mother, but I can understand that you might be wishing that I was', and then talk to and care for the patient in the motherly way that he is needing. However, if the patient persists with a misperception (or hallucination) and is distressed that he is not believed, it may be better to respond as if what he says is true. For instance a man who could not settle to sleep because of the 'rabbits under his bed', went to sleep contentedly when the nurse told him she had shut them up in their hutch for the night.

Some patients who have been through traumatic events in their past, re-live these in a vivid and terrifying way when they become seriously ill and their life is once again in danger. It is as if the person, in attempting to make sense of the present fear, remembers times when he experienced similar emotions, so that at least he recognizes his feelings as familiar. Thus, a woman who was afraid of death kept re-living times when her mother beat her severely as a child. As an old woman in hospital, she became afraid of the nurses, assuming they might do the same. Similarly, a man who had been torpedoed and watched others drowning all around him went through that experience over and over again as his own death approached years later. Patients like these can be helped by encouragement to talk about what really happened so that their distress can be shared and understood. Then, it is often possible for them to separate past and present, and to distinguish what is a terrible memory from what is happening now.

The conditions described so far are characterized by some degree of impairment of consciousness and should be included in the diagnostic category of acute confusional state or delirium. But other patients who are reported to be confused have a clear sensorium and behave inappropriately for quite different reasons. An example is early dementia in which there is impairment of short-term memory and loss of intellectual ability. These patients are disoriented because they cannot remember what has been said to them or where their bed is. It is important that the correct diagnosis be made because the patient's distress can be minimized by skilful management, even though it may be impossible to improve his mental function. Similarly patients who are hallucinating, paranoid, or deluded may also be mistakenly labelled confused because of their odd behaviour. All these conditions will be encountered from time to time as concomitants or complications of malignant disease, adding to the distress of the patient and his family and making good care more difficult than usual for the staff. Their diagnosis and management at home or in a general hospital setting will therefore be briefly discussed later in this chapter.

MEDICATION AS A CAUSE OF CONFUSION

The commonest cause of confusion in very ill patients is medication, and diagnostic assessment should begin with a review of all the drugs the patient is receiving. One reason for excessive medication is that, as symptoms worsen or new ones develop, prescribers tend to add new drugs or increase current ones without giving due consideration to cumulative effects and interactions. Night sedatives should not be used to procure sleep if a patient is being kept awake by a specific treatable cause, e.g. pain, anxiety, or insomnia due to depression. When drugs are given for any of these conditions, it may be appropriate to reduce or omit the current night sedative. On the other hand, sudden withdrawal of a drug that the patient has used for years, for example diazepam, a barbiturate, or alcohol, may also precipitate confusion.

When the introduction of a new drug is followed by confusion, it should be withdrawn, and if necessary a drug from a slightly different class substituted to see if improvement ensues. It should not be assumed that the cause of confusion cannot be medication that has been given for some time before the onset. The drug may have gradually reached toxic levels because of its long half-life (e.g. diazepam) or because the patient metabolizes and excretes it less effectively due to the progressive nature of his illness.

The filter model can usefully provide a way of thinking about how drugs cause confusion. Sedatives can be perceived as decreasing the permeability of the filter to stimuli from the environment so that less information is taken in. (In depression and anxiety also, and in severe pain, the patient is so preoccupied with his experience that stimuli from the outside world do not register. He may then appear disoriented, not knowing the time of day or where he is, and testing him may also reveal impairment of short-term memory. This syndrome should not be mistaken for early dementia, which it resembles. It is reversible if the underlying cause can be treated, and so the patient like this who is worried that he is becoming demented should be reassured.)

Stimulants increase the permeability of the filter so that signals are perceived as being more intense, and the patient over-reacts. Drugs which produce hallucinations, nightmares, paranoia and other psychotic states may act by increasing the permeability of the filter to unconscious material. The psychoses occasionally caused by steroids can be viewed in this way too. The whole picture of the acute brain syndrome or delirium can be viewed as a release phenomenon. There is a slackening of the control the patient usually maintains over the expression of his personality. The naturally timid person may become terrified, the slightly suspicious becomes paranoid, the anxious becomes agitated, and the depressed becomes suicidal. Unpleasant memories which have been suppressed, and the more primitive part of the unconscious which is usually inaccessible in health, may enter awareness and be expressed.

Table 2 is modified from the list in Davison's paper (Davison, 1981) on toxic psychosis which gives an excellent and detailed survey of this subject.

Table 2. Drugs inducing delirium.

Tranquillizers and hypnotics	Barbiturates Benzodiazepines Phenothiazines
Cardiotherapeutic drugs	Digoxin Diuretics β-blockers
Anticholinergic drugs	Atropine and homatropine Hyoscine Antiparkinsonian drugs Tricyclic antidepressants
Dopamine agonists	Levodopa Bromocriptine Amantadine hydrochloride
Antibiotics	Penicillin Streptomycin Sulphonamides
Anticonvulsants	Phenytoin Sodium valproate
Miscellaneous drugs	Morphine Disulfiram Piperazine Cimetidine Chloroquine Oral hypoglycaemic drugs
Drug withdrawal	Barbiturates Benzodiazepines Chlormethiazole Alcohol

Modified from Davison (1981).

Oncologists particularly need to know that a few patients on morphine (and rather more on pentazocine) experience unpleasant, mainly visual, hallucinations. Some patients are drowsy when treatment is initiated or if the dose is increased by more than the patient requires to control his pain. Conversely, if the analgesic requirement is suddenly diminished, e.g. by a successful nerve block, and the morphine dose is not reduced, toxic effects may occur. Other drugs which cause problems include tricyclic antidepressants which may produce agitation, especially in the elderly, and some β-blockers (especially propranolol), which produce vivid dreams and hallucinations. Some or all of the phenomena of confusion are produced by antiparkinsonian drugs (especially benzhexol hydrochloride), anticonvulsants (especially phenytoin), anti-inflammatory drugs (especially indomethacin), and cimetidine. Steroids do not cause a true delirium but they may induce a euphoric mental state which rarely proceeds to hypomania. More commonly they cause depression or a paranoid state. When psychosis supervenes in a patient with a brain tumour who is being treated with dexamethasone, the clinician is faced with a dilemma as the mental state could be caused by the tumour itself, by the dexamethasone, or it could be the patient's response to the stressful recognition that he has a terminal malignant disease. There is no easy way of distinguishing these three and treatment has to be empirical, using haloperidol in a crisis to control the psychosis while the effect of dexamethasone reduction is assessed.

OTHER CAUSES OF CONFUSION

Most items in Table 3 are self-explanatory. Occasionally patients with advanced malignant disease in whom an intercurrent infection occurs are wrongly diagnosed as suffering from a terminal delirium. The referring doctor may be surprised when such a patient recovers and lives for a further few months. Similarly, how actively a condition like hypercalcaemia should be treated depends on the extent of the underlying condition. If the patient has other problems that have made life scarcely worth living, the hypercal-

Table 3. Causes of confusion.

Medication	most drugs acting on the CNS; steroids
Infection	whether pyrexial or not
Trauma	head injury; subdural haematoma
Tumour	cerebral primary or secondaries; malignant disease elsewhere
Cerebrovascular disease	strokes; dementia
Cardiac and respiratory failure	Anoxia; hypercapnia
Biochemical and metabolic	electrolyte imbalance (dehydration, hyponatraemia, hypokalaemia); hypocalcaemia; uraemia; hepatic failure; hypoglycaemia
General discomfort	Full bladder or bowel; uncomfortable bedding; pruritus
Emotional stress	Facing death

caemia can be regarded as a terminal event and its effects treated symptomatically; but if the patient has been reasonably well, active treatment should be attempted.

Patients and relatives are sometimes relieved to be told that the cause of the confusion is medication, a change in blood chemistry, or even a tumour. These conditions do not carry a stigma in the way that inexplicable insanity does. Some patients, for at least part of the time, can separate out the ideas 'Myself' and 'My illness'. They are helped to do this if, in a lucid interval, they are reassured by remarks like 'Whatever strange things your tumour or illness makes you say or do, we know that you yourself are alright'. When delirium is part of the process of dying, it comforts some families to be told that in many illnesses death comes slowly, with some systems failing before others. For the patient who has a major cerebro-vascular accident or heart attack, everything stops at once. In the case of their relative it is not that he has gone mad, but only that his brain, which is a very delicate organ, is dying a little faster than other parts of his body.

Stress has been included in the list because, for a few patients, the sudden realization that they have a terminal illness or that their condition has got dramatically worse is so disturbing that they respond with a short-lived psychogenic confusional state or psychosis. This is recognizable by its timing and by the absence of other precipitants. It usually clears within a few days as the patient either comes to terms with what is happening or copes with it by denial.

TREATMENT

Hallucination and misperception

Treatment depends on accurate diagnosis and it is particularly important to distinguish between the patient who is hallucinating and the one who is misperceiving. The latter is misinterpreting a stimulus, usually a sound, which is really there. For instance, a farmer's wife who was drowsy thought the vaccum cleaner she could hear outside her room was a milking machine, and said she must get up to attend to the cows. The nurse who was with her reported that she was hallucinating, but treatment which would have been appropriate for hallucinations (haloperidol or chlorpromazine) would have sedated her further and probably made her worse. Instead she needed to be moved to a quieter place until the cause of her drowsiness could be reversed.

Hallucinations are sensory experiences without external stimuli. A visual or auditory memory that would normally be unconscious is released into awareness; or a sensory area of the brain is stimulated, for example by a tumour, producing phenomena like those of temporal lobe epilepsy. Treatment should be aimed at suppression of the abnormal experience, either with haloperidol or a phenothiazine derivative. In the case of hallucinations related to a tumour, an anticonvulsant may be more effective. In delirium (especially that due to alcohol withdrawal) there may be a more mixed picture; clouding of consciousness increases the liability to misperception, and hallucinations and disturbances of behaviour in response to these may occur at the same time. Such a person settles best when cared for by staff with whom he is familiar, in a well-lit quiet room. Small amounts of sedation, by making him more drowsy, may increase his confusion. If he is too disturbed to be quietened by reassurance, heavy sedation may be required until the cause of the problem has been treated. Unfortunately, this may silence the shouting and make the patient too unco-ordinated to run away, without relieving the mental turmoil, as evinced by the frowning and rapid eye movements of someone having distressing dreams.

The use of drugs

The importance of reducing or stopping any unnecessary drugs has already been emphasized. The specific syndromes of hallucinosis and paranoia are best treated with haloperidol. In the physically ill and the elderly, 1.5 mg two or three times daily may suffice. In the more robust patient, treatment should begin with 5 mg two or three times daily. Emergencies such as mania may require intramuscular injection of haloperidol 10 mg every two hours until control is achieved, changing to the oral route and reducing the dose as soon as the acute phase subsides. Parkinsonian side-effects are seldom encountered when haloperidol is used in this way, and anticholinergic drugs (e.g. orphenadrine hydrochloride) should only be added if the dose reduction is ineffective, or in the rare emergency of an acute dystonic reaction. Chlorpromazine is preferable only if its sedative effect is needed to enable the patient to sleep until the mental turmoil is relieved. The slurring of speech and the drowsiness which it produces add to some patients' distress. An initial dose of chlorpromazine 100 mg in tablet or syrup form, or 100 mg by deep intramuscular injection may be repeated 6-hourly until control is achieved. Chlorpromazine suppositories may also be used. Occasionally very disturbed patients need a much larger dose—up to 1 g in 24 hours. Postural hypotension is the foremost complication, and patients on high doses must be kept in bed, at least initially. When chlorpromazine is being used to control a very disturbing psychotic state, the dose level should be determined by the mental state (e.g. speech content, facial expression, eye movements) and not only by the level of consciousness. A long sleep after a large dose does not necessarily mean that too much was used. The patient may have been exhausted by his terrifying experiences and may need to sleep to recover. The side-effect of sedation is no more relevant in determining the right dose of antipsychotic drug in psychosis than it is in determining the dose of analgesic to be used for pain control.

Anxiety and agitation not associated with hallucinations or psychosis are best treated with diazepam, where sedation is an advantage, or clobazam where it is not. Agitated depression will require an antidepressant. The management of these conditions is described in Chapter 8. Toward the very end of life, diamorphine and hyoscine hydrobromide together may be more effective than anything else in producing a tranquil state. The dose of diamorphine will usually be determined by the level of this drug or morphine previously required by the patient, and it can be combined with 400–800 μg of hyoscine hydrobromide, both drugs being repeated every four hours.

RECOGNIZING AND MANAGING DEMENTIA

Early dementia may be missed in patients suffering from malignant disease simply because it has not been thought of. Where memory loss leads to disorientation or disinhibition allows lapses in social behaviour and lack of modesty, the patient may be mistakenly labelled confused. If he ceases to read or watch television or she no longer does the complicated knitting she once enjoyed, it is often assumed that depression is the cause. (Depression can also be a reaction to awareness of early dementia, and so co-exist with it.) A few simple tests such as asking a patient to remember (and recall after 5 minutes) an address and the name of three objects, or your own name, often reveals a surprising deficit in people who are well able to maintain a social façade. Cognitive impairment can be shown up by asking about recent problems in paying bills etc., and checked by getting the patient to do simple calculations. His initial embarrassment at having his impairment discovered is usually more than compensated for if he is treated with sympathetic understanding, especially if he has become increasingly aware of his declining powers and been frightened about what will eventually happen as a result. The explanation that this change in him is not his fault but may be associated with his disease, brings relief. Explaining the situation to the family is helpful too. (A patient like this used to 'mind the phone' for her husband's business when her malignant disease made her no longer able to help him more actively in their shop. He became angry and she became upset when messages were forgotten or confused, and both of them thought she had 'gone stupid'. As soon as he understood what was wrong he became sympathetic and she felt much better when demands which had become inappropriate were no longer made on her.)

A patient may be able to compensate for early dementia while in good health and familiar surroundings. The combination of illness, medication, and transfer to hospital may tip the balance. Such patients may revert almost to their former competence if they can be nursed as much as possible by familiar people and return home at the earliest opportunity. When improvement is not possible, good management aims to minimize the occasions when the patient is distressed by confrontation with his disability. To greet him by saying something like 'I expect you remember that I am the doctor who talked to you yesterday about the injection I am going to give you . . .' saves him having to hide the fact that he cannot recall the people and events of the preceding day.

UNDERSTANDING AND MANAGING PARANOID REACTIONS

Paranoia may be caused by medication such as steroids or bromocriptine. It may also be the result of a patient using the mental mechanism of projection when he cannot bear the stress of knowing that his illness has got suddenly worse or is likely to lead to his death. It is so much less threatening to be convinced that the cause of the problem is outside one's self and so can be dealt with effectively by taking action of one kind or another. Thus, 'I am dying' becomes 'Someone is plotting to kill me' or, more symbolically, 'Someone is stealing my money.' The delusional belief that medication is the cause of deterioration leads some patients to refuse drugs that they need, even for pain relief. Occasionally patients who are very ill but want to discharge themselves use the same mechanism. One such man said: 'I wasn't as ill as this when I was at home. It must be this place that is making me worse.' Sometimes a person like this can be helped to understand that it is really the progress of the illness that is making them so afraid. If they can admit this and accept comfort, the paranoia ceases. Others are angered by such an approach and will only respond to a drug such as haloperidol. Giving medication to a paranoid patient can be difficult. To disguise it is unwise, as they are often very alert, and discovery of the ruse would only serve to confirm their suspicions. They may accept something 'to calm their nerves' from a member of staff they know well and trust, or often from a member of their family. Once it has taken effect they may be more prepared to talk about and acknowledge their true situation, and the medication may be gradually discontinued.

Taking care over the diagnosis and management of confused patients is well worthwhile. Their suffering and that of their families is reduced, and others in the vicinity benefit too, including the staff. In situations where indiscriminate sedation might otherwise have been used, understanding brings increased interest and confidence in handling patients who are potentially very disturbing or disturbed.

Acknowledgements

Much of this chapter is taken from *Facing Death: Patients, Families and Professionals* by A. Stedeford (1984). London: Heinemann Medical Books.

REFERENCES

Davison K (1981) Toxic psychosis. *British Journal of Hospital Medicine* **26**(5): 530–537.
Stedeford A (1984) *Facing Death: Patients, Families and Professionals*. London: Heinemann Medical Books.

8

Anxiety and depression

JENNIFER HUGHES

At least 25% of patients receiving treatment for cancer become anxious or depressed to an extent which adds a significant extra burden to their physical suffering (Plumb and Holland, 1977; Derogatis et al, 1983; Bukberg et al, 1984).

In their pure forms, anxiety and depression are separate entities, but many patients develop features of both these mood states in combination.

SYMPTOMATOLOGY

Mood

A disturbance of mood is the central symptom. The anxious patient is troubled by constant worry, fear or dread, so that relaxation is impossible. The depressed patient feels low, miserable, pessimistic and hopeless. All interest and enthusiasm is lost, so life seems pointless and empty. Some depressed patients feel so guilty and worthless that they regard themselves as unfit to live. Suicide is a real risk in such cases. Daily activities are disrupted because the patient cannot concentrate, or cannot summon the energy or interest to do anything.

In some cases the mood disturbance makes the patient hostile, sullen, irritable or aggressive, and it is easy to dismiss such patients as unpleasant unco-operative people, whereas sympathetic inquiry might reveal that this behaviour is not typical of their usual personality.

Sleep

Sleep is usually disturbed in both anxious and depressed patients. Anxiety often delays the onset of sleep for several hours, then if and when sleep does come, its quality is unsatisfying, being interrupted by unpleasant dreams or episodes of panic causing sudden wakefulness. In depression, the classical sleep pattern is early morning waking, in which the patient can get off to sleep normally in the early part of the night but wakes for good in the small hours. Depressed mood in such cases is often at its worst before dawn, and undergoes a gradual improvement as the day goes on. This characteristic pattern of early morning waking and diurnal variation of mood provides a useful diagnostic marker for depressive illness, although there are many depressed patients who do not show this sleep pattern. Some complain of sleep disturbance during an earlier stage of the night, and others sleep longer and more heavily than usual but still wake up tired.

Physical symptoms

Physical (somatic) symptoms are usually present in both anxious and depressed patients. Quite often these form the patient's presenting complaints, and changes in mood and sleep pattern are only elicited if the right questions are asked. Poor appetite and weight loss are usually found with both anxiety and depression, but a minority of patients eat for comfort and gain weight. The patient often feels generally unwell, with mental and physical tiredness, muscular tension or pain, and constant fatigue. In anxiety, disturbance of the autonomic nervous system can give rise to numerous specific physical symptoms. Tremor, sweating, palpitations, headaches, shortness of breath, dysphagia, nausea, diarrhoea, and frequency of micturition are common ones. Individual patients may be badly affected by one of these symptoms but do not complain of the others.

AETIOLOGY

Neurochemical disturbance

There is laboratory evidence of neurochemical disturbances in the more severe forms of mood disturbance; for example monoamine neurotransmitter systems involving noradrenaline and 5-hydroxytryptamine (5-HT) are disturbed in patients with depression. A direct association between depression and cancer, presumably mediated by some physiological effect of the tumour, has sometimes been reported, for example in pancreatic cancer (Fras et al, 1967; Holland et al, 1986); but this phenomenon has not been explained and its importance remains uncertain. In clinical terms, anxiety and depression usually are better understood as a result of interaction between personal predisposition and environmental stress.

Predisposition to mood disturbance

Genetic predisposition to both anxiety and depression has been demonstrated by twin studies and adoption studies. Personality characteristics, which are shaped partly by inheritance and partly by environment in early life, also help to determine vulnerability to anxiety and depression.

Patients who have a family history of psychiatric illness or suicide, have required psychiatric treatment themselves in the past, have shown extreme reactions to previous crisis in their lives, or whose personalities are described as sensitive, dependent, 'neurotic' or highly strung, are probably more at risk of becoming seriously anxious or depressed if they develop cancer than are their more psychologically robust counterparts. However, there are plenty of exceptions to this general statement. Some apparently vulnerable patients are able to mobilize hidden reserves when they develop cancer, and do not become anxious or depressed, whereas other cancer patients unexpectedly break down for the first time in their lives.

The stress of the physical illness

Many aspects of having cancer can induce anxiety or depression. For some patients, one isolated aspect seems to be the chief cause of their distress.

Knowing the diagnosis is the worst blow for some. The word 'cancer' still carries a stigma, as for one middle-aged woman with breast cancer who commented 'I couldn't tell anybody what I'd got . . . I was so ashamed. I felt like a leper.' Cancer also implies pain, disfigurement, and a hopeless prognosis. Many patients, though they do know their diagnosis, take pains to avoid having to say the word cancer. Some patients, even nowadays, do not know their diagnosis, but many of these suspect it and feel anxious and depressed as a result. They are unable to talk openly with their doctors, who usually have their own psychological barriers about discussing cancer, and consequently it is impossible for a trusting and supportive doctor–patient relationship to develop. Presumably problems such as these will become less common in future now that cancer is more freely discussed, and improvements in long-term survival are publicized.

Uncontrolled physical symptoms like pain, breathlessness or nausea can make patients anxious and depressed. Even if specific symptoms like these are well controlled, the weakness and general debility caused by advanced cancer may cause depression. 'Not being able to do things' was considered the worst aspect of their illness by over half of one series of patients admitted for continuing care (Hughes and Lee, 1987). To a large extent, distress from this source is unavoidable, but sometimes it is possible to suggest new ways for patients to continue their former activities, or find alternatives which are reasonably satisfying. An occupational therapist could advise in such cases.

Treatment for cancer may cause anxiety and depression too. Disfigurement or functional loss, resulting from cancer operations like mastectomy or colostomy, prove psychological disasters for some patients, though others take them in their stride. Most patients dislike chemotherapy, and anxiety before a new course of injections begins is extremely common. Similarly, anticipation of radiotherapy provokes anxiety for some. Depression following treatment occurs with both chemotherapy and radiotherapy, sometimes because of an identifiable side-effect like hair loss or vomiting, sometimes probably due to a direct effect on mood. Some patients are not specifically upset by cancer treatments, but simply say they dread hospitals, anaesthetics, or injections. Though some treatments tend to be more generally acceptable than others, there are no rules about which regimes cause least distress. Discussion with individual patients is the only way to discover what treatment regime will suit their particular preferences. For example, contrary to the expectations of many doctors, a significant minority of women with breast cancer elect to have a mastectomy rather than a 'lumpectomy' if given the choice. Sometimes patients are averse to certain treatments because they have misconceptions about them; for example some people believe that radiotherapy is only used for patients who are shortly going to die, or that it will make them permanently radioactive and a danger to their family. Providing information leaflets to patients about to embark on new treatments is an acceptable and economical way to dispel the more common fears.

Some patients are more concerned for their relatives' welfare than about their own condition. Patients may be uncertain how much to tell relatives about the illness, and family discussion on the subject is often inhibited. There may be practical worries about the future of frail spouses, or dependent children, for whose care the patient has been responsible. Financial difficulties may arise if the family member with cancer can no longer earn money, or when the illness demands expenses like extra heating or frequent travel to hospital. Social case-work can help to resolve both emotional and practical problems for families as a whole.

Other life events and social difficulties

Anxiety and depression in the general population are often associated with recent 'life events' such as bereavement, or chronic social difficulties such as an unhappy marriage. The same is true for cancer patients. Many of those who are anxious or depressed attribute these feelings to factors other than their own physical illness, and may report that the mood disorder began before the cancer was even suspected. One widow said 'My husband's death was the start of my depression. The breast cancer was nothing, compared with losing him.'

DIFFERENTIAL DIAGNOSIS

'Normal' reactions to stress versus 'pathological' mood disorder

To some extent, of course, anxiety and depression are natural and appropriate reactions to having cancer. A few cancer patients do not admit to either emotion, some being able to accept their illness calmly from the start and others seeming unaware there is anything seriously wrong, but most cancer patients do feel anxious and depressed at some stage of their illness. Some of these are experiencing a 'normal' reaction and others a 'pathological' mood disorder. 'Normal' reactions last for days or weeks, rather than for a month or more, and they do not become so severe as to dominate the patient's life. These reactions are readily understandable as a response to circumstances, and in some cases they probably fulfil a useful function by advancing the process of psychological adaptation to the physical illness. They do not require treatment by formal psychotherapy or psychotropic drugs, but the distress they cause can be kept to a minimum by observing a few simple rules of good clinical practice. These include establishing warm staff–patient relationships, providing adequate time for patients to discuss their illness, giving them as much information as they wish to have, and avoiding needless delays in investigation and treatment.

The boundary between normal reaction and pathological mood change is not clear-cut. The difference is partly one of degree, that is how severe and long-lasting the changes are. There is also a qualitative difference. Patients with a clinical depression often describe their mood change as different in kind from ordinary sadness, and they may seem to experience a change in personality, feeling guilty or worthless and no longer able to take pleasure in anything at all. In contrast, cancer patients who are not clinically depressed usually continue to appreciate life even when they are terminally ill, still being able to value the company of relatives, friends or pets, and to enjoy physically undemanding pursuits like reading or listening to music. Cancer patients who are not depressed seldom contemplate suicide, even if their disease is incurable, surprising though this may seem.

The difference between normal reaction and pathological mood change is well summarized in the paper by Plumb and Holland (1977): 'The self-esteem of the typical advanced cancer patient . . . is relatively intact. The patient may loathe his situation but does not loathe himself.'

The spectrum from 'not depressed' through 'normal depressive reaction' to 'pathological depression' can be illustrated by quotations from a series of patients who were asked to describe their mood just after being admitted for terminal care (Hughes and Lee, 1987):

> 'I keep quite happy really.'
> 'I'm a cheerful little soul.'
> 'I feel quite cheerful—it isn't any good going round with a long face my dear—there's plenty worse off than me!'
> 'I do knitting, I like reading, my son takes me out in the car, so I feel quite cheerful really.'
> 'I won't let it get me down. No, I've been feeling quite cheerful.'
> 'I've learnt to accept the condition I've got and I don't get depressed about it much—only in the mornings when I see the sun but I can't go out and enjoy it.'
> 'I'm alright—I try not to let it get me down—I've got to accept it, haven't I.'
> 'I get a bit depressed when I think of the future, but I try to keep cheerful.'
> 'I try to look on the bright side of things, but how can you not be a bit depressed when you're ill.'
> 'I try to keep a brave face but I do get down sometimes, yes.'
> 'I do get depressed occasionally—frustrated rather than depressed, because I can't do things.'
> 'Yes, I get a bit depressed you know, it's being on my own and having to cope alone.'
> 'I'm feeling very depressed. I've been weeping and feeling really, really down. I can't get out to do my work any more you see. And I lost my husband six years ago.'
> 'I've been feeling depressed and low-spirited lately. It's my illness—you know damn well there's nothing you can do for me.'
> 'I've nothing to be cheerful about . . . I've lost my wife, I've lost my health . . . it's all been terrible . . . there's no point in living.'

Symptoms of cancer or other physical disease

The mental symptoms of mood disorder can be part of an organic brain syndrome caused by the complications of the tumour or its treatment. In such cases, some degree of mental confusion is often found as well as anxiety or depression. The causes of these syndromes fall into three groups:

1. Cerebral metastases, or primary brain tumours.
2. Metabolic disturbances, e.g. uraemia, respiratory failure, hypercalcaemia.
3. Treatment effects. Drugs such as corticosteroids and some cytotoxics can cause mood disturbance. Radiotherapy often appears to cause depression, though how far this is due to a physical effect on the brain is unknown.

The physical symptoms of mood disorder such as anorexia, weight loss, fatigue and pain are indistinguishable from the systemic symptoms of malignant disease.

Besides cancer, many other physical disorders can mimic anxiety and depression. The classic example is thyroid disease: the symptoms of thyrotoxicosis are similar to those of anxiety, and the symptoms of hypothyroidism are similar to those of depression. Many other examples exist.

Diagnostic mistakes in either direction are easily made unless both psychiatric and physical diagnoses are considered, and the history, examination and investigation covers both. Delays in appropriate treatment can result:

> A man in his 60s consulted his family doctor complaining of tiredness and general malaise. He was treated with diazepam for several months before physical investigations were performed. He was then found to have lung cancer.

> A woman in her 50s developed headaches, poor appetite and loss of weight, a year after mastectomy for breast cancer. She was thought to have cerebral metastases but her brain scan was normal. Questioning revealed the classic symptoms of depressive illness and she responded well to a course of amitriptyline.

MANAGEMENT

Recognition

The first step in managing mood disorders is to recognize their presence. Anxiety and depression are not always obvious. Many patients are reluctant to complain about psychological symptoms, either because they feel ashamed of them, or because they assume staff in cancer treatment units are only interested in physical symptoms, or because they themselves do not realize their symptoms are mental rather than physical in origin. Screening of all patients, by means of self-rating questionnaires such as the *General Health Questionnaire* (Goldberg, 1986) or the *Hospital Anxiety and Depression Scale* (Zigmond and Snaith, 1983), is one way to detect cases of mood disorder, but such questionnaires are probably more useful in research than for clinical practice. They are not a substitute for clinical assessment; for example they do not distinguish between an acute but self-limiting emotional crisis and a sustained mood disorder which merits treatment.

Staff–patient relationships

Essential to good management are the kind of staff–patient relationships which permit emotional problems to be disclosed and followed through. In the setting of the continuous personal support which good staff–patient relationships provide, it becomes easier for patients to raise the queries and difficulties which arise at various stages of their illness. Milder cases of anxiety and depression will resolve, or be prevented in the first place, if all patients are given the opportunity to talk about the illness, having their questions answered adequately and being able to express their main concerns. Ideally, the staff providing this service should be doctors or nurses senior enough to have a wide knowledge of the condition concerned, mature and well-adjusted enough to discuss emotional issues, and in a position to take an on-going part in the patient's care. Patients value continuity of staff, and find frequent changes of personnel disruptive.

Barriers to this kind of supportive staff–patient relationship may arise from either side. Some staff ignore patients' efforts to discuss emotional problems especially when, as often happens, the patient broaches them in some indirect way. Other staff deal with them inappropriately. Some telling clinical examples from a terminal care setting are given by Maguire (1985). One common form of inappropriate response is trying to 'jolly patients along' instead of acknowledging and respecting their distress. Giving false promises like 'you'll feel better tomorrow' or advice like 'cheer up and look on the bright side' is usually unhelpful. Another type of inappropriate response involves leaping to false conclusions about what is wrong, instead of listening to patients' real concerns, for example assuming that tearfulness is due to pain when it is really about fear of dying. In order to respond more effectively, staff need to be aware of their own and their patients' feelings, and this can often be achieved through regular group meetings for staff, perhaps using teaching techniques like role-play and video. Highly sophisticated psychological awareness is not required to make this work, but a willingness to be flexible and honest is important. Introducing such a group in a traditional medical setting often inspires alarm and suspicion. There will be some staff who cannot or will not participate and some of these would probably be better placed in some other specialty. The current trend in many units, however, is veering in the opposite direction, and this has its dangers too; staff sometimes get carried away by the psychological approach to the extent that they neglect their patients' physical problems, or imagine psychological difficulties where none exist!

When mood disorders do develop and persist despite attention to these general guidelines on good staff–patient relationships, as in some cases they inevitably will, specific treatment is indicated and this may be psychological, physical, or a combination of the two.

Psychological treatments

The psychological treatments entail devoting regular amounts of time, traditionally one hour a week, to discussion about emotional issues. A simplified summary of the main approaches is given here.

Counselling involves giving information and advice about the patient's illness, and considering its emotional consequences. This should ideally happen anyway in the course of ordinary staff–patient relationships, as discussed above, but counselling puts the matter on a more formal basis, and involves more detailed and prolonged discussion than usually takes place during 'routine' care. Counselling for cancer patients is often provided by specialist nurses and/or by volunteers who have themselves received treatment for cancer. Group counselling, in which the interaction is with other patients rather than with professional carers, is the most helpful type of intervention for some.

Psychotherapy of the psychodynamic type involves exploring patients' feelings and behaviour at a deeper level than is intended in counselling. The process involves considering how current problems may be derived from past experience in other spheres of life, increasing patients' awareness of feelings or memories which were too painful for them to acknowledge spontaneously, and the analysis of interpersonal relationships including that between the patient and the therapist. Many schools of psychotherapy exist and they may be practised by a psychiatrist or other suitably trained professional. Few cancer patients require formal psychodynamic psychotherapy though it may occasionally be indicated in the complex case, providing the patient is physically robust enough to undergo a course of treatment which lasts several months and may well be emotionally painful or challenging.

More recently developed types of psychological treatment, for example the *behaviour therapies*, are less concerned with uncovering the origins of symptoms, but focus on their everyday management, through devising individually tailored active methods of helping the patient face a feared situation, or banish thinking patterns which perpetuate depression or anxiety. Patients are given practical exercises, for example a graded programme of encounters with a feared object or situation. Relaxation exercises are often taught as an accompaniment. This type of treatment was developed by clinical psychologists, but may be practised by psychiatrists or psychiatric nurses who are trained in the techniques.

Counselling is offered to all patients attending for cancer treatment in some centres, especially for breast cancer patients although their need is not necessarily greater than that of patients with other types of malignancy. A review of research studies gauging the efficacy of counselling (Watson, 1983) concludes that the effects are generally beneficial, but not all patients want to take part. Sometimes the psychological benefit is not direct, but arises because counselling enables depressed and anxious patients to be recognized and treated at an early stage. Occasionally counselling might precipitate mood disorder, rather than prevent it, through increasing patients' conscious awareness of the gravity of their disease and preventing them from 'denying' their condition or, in the case of group counselling, through bringing them into contact with similar patients who are not progressing well. These problems do not seem to arise very often, provided the counsellor is skilled.

Physical treatments

Severely depressed or anxious patients usually require some form of physical treatment, i.e. psychotropic drugs or electroconvulsive therapy (ECT), in addition to a psychological approach.

Antidepressants

Antidepressant drugs do not help unhappiness or distress, as opposed to depressive illness, and this is why the differentiation of transient stress reactions from sustained mood disorders is clinically important.

A standard antidepressant drug is the tricyclic amitriptyline, which has useful sedative properties and is therefore especially suitable for depressed patients with prominent sleep disturbance, agitation or anxiety. Amitriptyline has the disadvantage that side-effects, many attributable to its anticholinergic properties, are common: dry mouth, dizziness on standing due to postural hypotension, and drowsiness being most often found. Such side-effects tend to be worst in the first few days of treatment, whereas the antidepressant benefits are usually delayed two weeks or more, so it is important for both patient and doctor to persevere with the drug for a reasonable period. More serious side-effects, which may be considered contraindications to amitriptyline in the physically frail, include cardiac conduction defects, urinary retention, constipation, and precipitation of glaucoma. The starting dose of amitriptyline may be 50 mg or 75 mg daily in a reasonably fit patient, though old or frail subjects may do better to start with 25 mg or even just 10 mg. If tolerated satisfactorily, the drug should be increased to the limit of tolerance which may be up to 250 mg daily. When the drug fails to improve depressed mood, this is often because it has been given in too low a dose for too short a time. Giving the total dose at night is often most satisfactory, being easy for the patient to remember, and providing maximum hypnotic effect.

Though amitriptyline is one of the oldest antidepressant drugs it remains the first choice for many psychiatrists. If amitriptyline proves ineffective or difficult to tolerate, however, there are many other tricyclic antidepressants, and newer drugs of related structure, which may prove better for individual patients. The selection is to some extent a matter of trial and error but some guidelines exist as to which profile of depressive symptoms responds best to which drug. Another group of antidepressants is the monoamine oxidase inhibitors (MAOIs), for example phenelzine sulphate. MAOIs are seldom used as the first line of treatment, especially for physically ill patients, because of their myriad interactions with other drugs, including analgesics and anaesthetic agents. They may, however, be dramatically effective for certain depressions which are resistant to tricyclics. Flupenthixol is another compound which might be considered.

When both anxiety and depression are present in the same patient, the best strategy is usually to prescribe an antidepressant drug which has sedative properties. Many doctors fail to do this and choose an anxiolytic or hypnotic drug, which will not help the depressive element, and may do more harm than good in the long-term.

Anxiolytic and hypnotic drugs

Anxiolytic and hypnotic drugs are considered together because most compounds in current use for either purpose belong to the benzodiazepine family, and, although they tend to be marketed for one purpose or the other, they are to some extent interchangeable. The same drug is often an effective hypnotic when given in one large dose at night, and an effective anxiolytic when given in smaller doses by day. Widely used members of the group include diazepam and lorazepam for anxiety, and temazepam for insomnia.

Benzodiazepines. These are effective and cause few obvious side-effects in most patients, but there has been a recent backlash against them, due to the recognition that they are not so innocuous as once assumed. After more than a week or so of regular use, tolerance may develop, and so a larger dose is needed. Especially with a large dose there may be side-effects: sometimes obvious drowsiness or uncoordination, sometimes a more subtle lethargy and numbing of emotion. A minority of patients develop marked dependence on benzodiazepines, with flagrant withdrawal symptoms if they are stopped. Publicity about the potential adverse effects of diazepam (Valium) has turned many members of the public against drugs of this kind. Nevertheless, benzodiazepines may be very effective for short-term use and should not necessarily be avoided at all costs. Some of their potential side-effects are irrelevant for the patient with advanced cancer who is limited to sedentary activities and has not long to live. When anxiety is related to a specific situation, for example chemotherapy injections, anxiolytic drugs should be given before the patient is due to encounter the situation in question, rather than given daily on a regular dose schedule.

Tranquillizers. The 'major tranquillizers', like chlorpromazine and trifluoperazine hydrochloride, may also be used for treating anxiety. They may be more suitable than benzodiazepines for patients with advanced cancer who require sedation, and the anti-emetic properties of some drugs in this group also make them useful when nausea co-exists.

β-blockers. β-blocking drugs like propranolol are the first choice when the somatic symptoms of anxiety are more prominent than the psychological ones.

Electroconvulsive therapy

ECT is mainly used to treat severe depression; it involves passing a small electric current across the brain while the patient is under brief general anaesthesia. A 'course' of ECT involves repeating this procedure several times, usually every two or three days, to give an average of six treatments. Though ECT tends to inspire revulsion and fear, it is safer than many forms of drug treatment, the mortality being negligible and the only common side-effect being a mild temporary confusion and loss of recent memory. Not many cancer patients become depressed enough to need ECT, for this treatment works best in the severe forms of depression, but the occasional depressed cancer patient may benefit a great deal from its use, and its rapid onset of action could be a special advantage for patients whose life expectancy is limited.

When to consult a psychiatrist

The availability of a psychiatric opinion, and the level of interest and skill regarding psychiatric disorder among the doctors providing physical care, clearly influence this question but there are general guidelines. Family doctors and oncologists should be able to recognize straightforward cases of depression and anxiety, carry out basic counselling, and prescribe first-line drug treatment. A psychiatrist should be consulted:

1. In cases of severe depression, which may be life-threatening because the patient is at risk of suicide, or refuses food and drink. Substantial doses of psychotropic drugs, ECT, and psychiatric hospitalization may be indicated.
2. When first-line drug treatment has failed.
3. When complex long-standing problems, often involving personality and relationship difficulties, as well as the current physical illness, suggest a need for formal psychotherapy.

PROGNOSTIC SIGNIFICANCE

The idea that mood and attitude exert a direct influence on cancer prognosis is an intriguing one, and does gain some support from published studies (Greer et al, 1979; Rogentine et al, 1979; Derogatis et al, 1983). Only cursory consideration of the topic is relevant here.

Most studies have found that patients who show a marked determination to overcome their disease enjoy longer survival times, or higher rates of cure, than those with a passive or helpless reaction. Broadly speaking, 'positive' attitudes seem to predict a good outcome whereas patients who show 'negative' emotions, or repress their emotions, tend to do badly.

No clear evidence has emerged to link either anxiety or depression with cancer prognosis. Display of these emotions could be labelled either 'positive' or 'negative' depending how the terms are defined!

The possibility that covert advanced disease could determine mental attitude can seldom be discounted, so caution is needed in interpreting studies of this kind.

Many patients are aware of this field of research and want to know how their emotional adjustment is likely to affect the outcome of their cancer. In my view, the correct answer at the present time is that nobody knows.

CASE HISTORY

The following extract from a research interview with a woman in her 60s, who had had a mastectomy for breast cancer four months previously, illustrates both depression and anxiety:

'I've felt depressed for years really . . . some days worse than others. Then I had this pain in my breast and it used to worry me and I used to keep going to the doctor's and he kept examining me and saying, "Well, there's nothing there." I felt I was being a nuisance. That made me feel down, made me feel depressed and wonder what's wrong. The doctor got fed up with me. Then one day I looked in the mirror and the breast had a big dent, so I thought right, I'm going back. And from then on it was really black. The doctor said I'll get you an appointment, but I couldn't have one that Monday because it was Bank Holiday, and I couldn't go the next Monday because there was a waiting list for the people who should've gone on Bank Holiday Monday so I had to wait another week—I had to wait three weeks to find what it was. I was fidgety, nervous, couldn't put my mind to anything while waiting to find out . . . and then to go and sit in that clinic . . . and then when I got up from the bed he said I think you've got cancer. He just said they'd take it off, take it all away . . . Now some days I'm very bad, very depressed.

I've been on sleeping tablets ten years . . . They help for a while but I wake up about three and I can't get back off, so I get up and have a cup of tea. When I was very bad and very down, after my operation, I slept less. I'd stay up till they'd all got to bed, as late as I could, but then about two I'd be awake again. The doctor said take two sleeping tablets, and I did, but I thought it's no good taking two if I'm not going to sleep any better. When you lie there and you can't sleep and everything's going round and round you think the worst.

I wasn't interested in anything after the op was done . . . it was all too much trouble . . . I got nothing done, I seemed slowed right down. But not relaxed. I was fidgety and restless all the time . . . picking and shredding things.

Because when the district nurse used to come, she said you've not had a lump, or a growth, or a tumour, you've had cancer. The specialist told me they'd cleared it all away so I said I've not got cancer, and she said once you've had it you can soon get it again, and that's got me worried about the other side, because I've had pain there like I had in this side. The district nurse that used to come here, you can't talk to her. I'd say it does hurt and she'd say, what do you expect after what you've had done. But I've been back to hospital three times and seen Sister X; she's very nice, very kind, you can talk to her, if you know what I mean.

Comment

This patient had chronic psychological and social problems dating back long before her breast cancer presented. She was unhappily married, had never settled down in the area where she lived and had experienced a string of bereavements over the past five years. With her background of chronic depression and poor personality adjustment, she was someone at high risk of developing psychological problems after having cancer diagnosed.

Poor staff–patient relationships stand out in her account. Her case has been chosen to illustrate the kind of avoidable difficulties which can arise, though it is fair to point out that she is an exception in this respect, and most other breast cancer patients treated in the same unit praise the treatment they have received. Her own personality and attitudes probably tended to alienate other people and make it difficult for them to establish a good relationship with her. Her family doctor, for example, may have failed to investigate her breast symptoms earlier because she had so often attended surgery with neurotic complaints. Neither the hospital doctor nor the district nurse seem to have been able to make any relationship with this patient but note that Sister X, the specialist nurse who is trained in counselling techniques, was able to do so.

The delay in her breast clinic appointment, which might have been avoided if NHS holidays were 'staggered', caused her much added distress.

The drug treatment of this patient could have been improved. Hypnotics given continuously for years tend to lose their effect, produce dependence, and cause side-effects. A course of antidepressant drugs would have been more appropriate.

Summary

A significant minority of cancer patients develop mood disorders, comprising anxiety or depression or a mixture of both. Distress over one or more aspects of the cancer is the obvious cause, but other social difficulties and adverse 'life events', and previous predisposition to psychiatric disorder, often contribute too. Many patients do not volunteer emotional problems spontaneously, so mood disorders are often missed unless regular inquiry about psychological symptoms is included in clinical assessment. Diagnostic difficulty may arise because the physical symptoms of mood disorder, especially depression, are similar to the symptoms of malignant disease, and the mental symptoms of mood disorder may be due to an organic brain syndrome secondary to complications of the cancer or its treatment.

Sympathetic discussion about the physical illness, within a supportive and continuing staff–patient relationship, may prevent or ameliorate some cases of mood disorder. More severe cases need specific additional treatment: psychotherapy, psychotropic drugs and occasionally ECT.

Whether anxiety and depression are related to the progress of the cancer itself is not clear, but there can be no doubt that unrecognized or untreated mood disorders add significantly to many cancer patients' suffering.

REFERENCES

Bukberg J, Penman D & Holland JC (1984) Depression in hospitalised cancer patients. *Psychosomatic Medicine* **46**(3): 199–212.

Derogatis LR, Morrow GR, Fetting J et al (1983) The prevalence of psychiatric disorders among cancer patients. *Journal of the American Medical Association* **249:** 751–757.

Fras I, Litin EM & Pearson JS (1967) Comparison of psychiatric symptoms in carcinoma of the pancreas with those in some other intra-abdominal neoplasms. *American Journal of Psychiatry* **123:** 1553–1562.

Goldberg D (1986) Use of the general health questionnaire in clinical work. *British Medical Journal* **293**(ii): 1188–1189.

Greer S, Morris T & Pettingale KW (1979) Psychological response to breast cancer: effect on outcome. *Lancet* **ii:** 785–787.

Holland JC, Korzun AH, Tross S et al (1986) Comparative psychological disturbance in patients with pancreatic and gastric cancer. *American Journal of Psychiatry* **143:** 982–986.

Hughes JE & Lee D (1987) Depressive symptoms in patients with terminal cancer. In Watson M & Greer S (eds) *Psychosocial Issues in Malignant Disease*. Oxford: Pergamon Press.

Maguire P (1985) Barriers to psychological care of the dying. *British Medical Journal* **291**(ii): 1711–1713.

Plumb MM & Holland J (1977) Comparative studies of psychological function in patients with advanced cancer. I. Self-reported depressive symptoms. *Psychosomatic Medicine* **39:** 264–276.

Rogentine GN et al (1979) Psychological factors in the prognosis of malignant melanoma: a prospective study. *Psychosomatic Medicine* **41:** 647–655.
Watson M (1983) Psychosocial intervention with cancer patients: a review. *Psychological Medicine* **13:** 839–846.
Zigmond AS & Snaith RP (1983) The hospital anxiety and depression scale. *Acta Psychiatrica Scandinavia* **67:** 361–370.

9

Bone pain

P. J. HOSKIN
G. W. HANKS

The skeleton is a common site for metastases to develop from a variety of primary tumours. Bone metastases are estimated to occur in 73% of patients dying from breast cancer, 32% of those with lung cancer and 85% of those with prostatic cancer (Abrams et al, 1950; Jacobs, 1983), and since these three sites alone account for approximately 40% of all patients with cancer, local bone pain and nerve compression pain caused by bone metastases are common problems. In a detailed analysis of the causes of pain in patients with advanced cancer, bone pain and nerve compression pain accounted for 38% of the pains detected (Twycross and Fairfield, 1982). The principle of management in patients with metastatic bone pain is careful analysis of individual sites of pain and their specific cause, on the basis of which rational treatment, individualized for each patient, can be instituted. In planning a treatment strategy it is important to consider both specific tumoricidal treatment and non-specific measures to control pain.

PATHOLOGY

Whilst direct invasion of bone by adjacent tumour may occur, skeletal metastases are usually the result of blood-borne dissemination of tumour cells. Tumour emboli take seed in the medullary cavity of the bone and only at a later stage is the cortex involved (Galasko, 1981). From studies of direct bone invasion in head and neck tumours (Carter, 1985) two phases of bone resorption in response to tumour cells have been described. Initially there is activation of osteoclasts causing bone resorption together with osteoblastic activity which results in focal production of osteoid and new bone. This is followed by a decline in osteoclastic activity, and tumour cells enter the areas of bone resorption and new bone formation. These processes are reflected in the familiar morphological features seen at post mortem and on X-ray, in which a combination of both bone destruction and new bone formation is invariably seen in association with bone metastases. The predominant picture of either lytic or sclerotic metastases on X-ray reflects the balance of these two processes; the finding of both lytic and sclerotic deposits within a single bone demonstrates the wide variation which can occur under apparently similar conditions. Pure lytic lesions, with no demonstrable new bone formation, are seen only in myeloma, the lymphomas and leukaemias (Galasko, 1981).

The factors controlling the initiation of this process in response to the presence of tumour cells are of considerable interest and have therapeutic implications. It seems likely that a chemical mediator is responsible for activating osteoclasts, but its precise nature remains unclear. Prostaglandins have been extensively investigated in this respect, and bone-resorbing activity can be clearly demonstrated in vitro for prostaglandins E_1, E_2, and $F_{1\alpha}$. Other non-prostaglandin osteolysins have also been demonstrated, including the lymphokine osteoclast activating factor (OAF), epidermal growth factor (EGF), and several other tumour-associated growth factors (Galasko, 1981; Carter, 1985). In vitro studies have demonstrated that both prostaglandin inhibitors such as indomethacin or ibuprofen and direct osteoclast inhibitors, in particular the diphosphonates, significantly reduce tumour-induced osteolysis (Powles, 1976; Galasko, 1981).

The underlying mechanism by which the process of tumour invasion results in bone pain remains poorly understood. It is a familiar clinical finding that one patient may have widespread bone metastases with little or no pain, whereas another may have only equivocal evidence for bone involvement by tumour, yet have severe pain. Thus the pathological process described above seems unlikely to account in itself for the pain with which it may be associated.

The cortex and medullary cavity are in general considered to be insensitive to pain though nerve fibres can be demonstrated in bone and its associated blood vessels. It is in the periosteum and joints where pain-sensitive nerve endings are found, and these peripheral nociceptors can be activated by both mechanical and chemical stimuli. The relative role in initiating the neuronal activity of distortion and increased pressure due to the growing tumour causing mechanical stimulation, and of chemical mediators such as prostaglandins, is unknown. Prostaglandins themselves do not produce pain (Horton, 1963) although they do sensitize peripheral nerve endings so that substances such as histamine and bradykinin can activate them and initiate pain transmission (Ferreira, 1972). There is also evidence to suggest that tumour shrinkage *per se* is not required to achieve relief from bone pain, since relief may be obtained with treatments which would not be expected to have a direct tumour-shrinking effect, such as hypophysectomy (Stoll, 1985), small single doses of radiotherapy (Price et al, 1986b), or calcitonin (Hindley, 1982).

MANAGEMENT OF BONE PAIN

Diagnosis

Whilst most bone pain occurring in patients with cancer will be related to metastatic disease, Twycross and Fairfield (1982) found that in 27% of patients admitted to a continuing care unit, musculoskeletal pain of non-malignant origin was present. An accurate diagnosis is therefore essential before initiating treatment. The presence of bone metastases may be suspected on the basis of the clinical history of pain in one of several bone sites, with associated tenderness, or radiation due to nerve root compression. Examination may reveal localized tenderness to percussion, local swelling, heat, or less frequently, a bruit at the site of a vascular metastasis. Simple investigations will generally confirm the presence of bone metastases in the presence of a clear history and physical findings. On occasions, however, pain may be less well localized and vague in nature with no abnormal findings on examination: more detailed investigations will then be required.

X-rays of the painful area will in many cases confirm the presence of bone metastases but their sensitivity is relatively poor (Edelstyn et al, 1967). Simple biochemical estimations reflecting bone turnover, such as serum alkaline and acid phosphatase, serum calcium, and urinary hydroxyproline/creatinine ratios, may provide further evidence for bone involvement by tumour. Where hepatic dysfunction is also suspected in the presence of a raised serum alkaline phosphatase, measurement of the specific bone isoenzyme will help clarify the situation.

Where plain X-rays are negative or equivocal, an isotope bone scan is the investigation of choice. In carcinomas of breast, bronchus and prostate, sensitivities of 87%, 97% and 99% respectively are reported for the detection of bone metastases using the isotope technetium (^{99m}Tc), with values of about 70% for melanoma, sarcoma, kidney and bladder (Goris and Bretille, 1985). For the common tumours, isotope scans represent the most sensitive method of detecting bone metastases. It is important to interpret results in the light of clinical findings and plain X-ray appearances in order to distinguish benign disease, usually degenerative or traumatic, from tumour invasion.

Only rarely will more sophisticated investigations be required to confirm the presence of bone metastases. Computerized tomography (CT) scanning may be considered for certain sites, in particular the spine, flat bones and sacrum, and is superior in demonstrating associated soft tissue infiltration (Sheedy et al, 1977; Cranston et al, 1984). This may be highly relevant in elucidating the mechanism of local pain in individual patients. The role of magnetic resonance imaging (MRI) in bone is currently under investigation. MRI appears to be superior to CT scanning in showing tumour in medullary cavity and surrounding soft tissues but less effective in detecting pathological fractures and areas of remineralization (Rimmer et al, 1985).

In phaeochromocytoma and neuroblastoma, scanning after administration of ^{131}I-labelled meta-iodo-benzyl guanidine (MIBG) will detect bone lesions not seen with conventional imaging. The use of isotope-tagged monoclonal antibodies for more common epithelial tumours is under investigation (Rainsbury et al, 1983).

Biopsy of a bone metastasis may be indicated where no primary site has been demonstrated, the patient presenting with bone pain and associated changes on X-ray or scan. Where the primary site is known and has been confirmed histologically, further tissue diagnosis of bone metastases is rarely necessary.

Pain assessment

Having confirmed the presence of metastatic bone disease in a site or sites consistent with the patient's pain, a more detailed pain assessment is essential before embarking upon treatment. Pain due to advanced cancer will in most cases have a prominent affective component. This means that in addition to the basic nociceptive input, the patient will exhibit a variable emotional response, incorporating amongst others anxiety, depression, fear and anger, which will modify their pain perception. Furthermore, it is unusual for a patient to have a single pain and it is important therefore to identify each individual pain, its site and likely cause, and also to consider their interrelationship. For example, a vertebral metastasis may cause not only local bone pain but also nerve root irritation and referred pain within the appropriate dermatome. Weakness and sensory loss due to nerve root compression may result in pressure sores, or involvement of sacral nerves may cause constipation or urinary dysfunction. Thus to consider the vertebral bone pain alone may be a misleading oversimplification of the overall pain which the patient is suffering. A careful assessment of the patient's physical condition together with consideration of their mental state will provide a basis for appropriate treatment.

Treatment

There are a number of treatment options available and it is important to consider the range of these at the outset. The three principal modalities of cancer treatment—radiotherapy, surgery and chemotherapy—may each have a role in selected cases in association with the use of appropriate analgesics and co-analgesic drugs.

Analgesics

In the majority of patients with pain due to advanced cancer the use of regular analgesic drugs will be the mainstay of their management. The basic principles governing analgesic use in this situation are to give the drug on a regular basis, preventing pain rather than treating each recurrence, and to use a drug of appropriate analgesic strength in an adequate dose. This means in practice that three main groups of analgesics are used for mild, moderate and severe pain, choosing one drug from each as shown in Figure 1 and selecting specific adjuvant therapies as appropriate. If a drug given regularly in adequate dosage fails to control pain, it is rarely useful to change to an alternative drug of similar strength, for example from coproxamol to dihydrocodeine. Rather this is an indication to reassess the pain, consider alternative co-analgesics or increase analgesia by moving up the analgesic ladder to a stronger drug. In order to evaluate changes in therapy it is best to make only one change at any one time. In this way, unnecessary medication is avoided and optimum pain control achieved in the most efficient way.

Mild pain. Patients presenting with scattered musculoskeletal pains may not require strong analgesics, and in all such patients who have not received

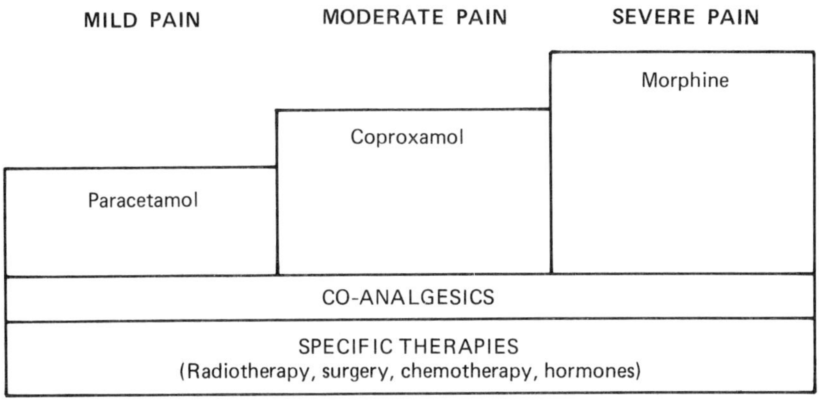

Figure 1. Principles of analgesic use.

regular medication with a simple analgesic this is the initial treatment of choice. Paracetamol or aspirin both have similar potency as simple analgesics and are the recommended drugs in this group. Paracetamol tends to be better tolerated than aspirin, which may be associated with a high incidence of gastro-intestinal side-effects (Hanks, 1983), and for this reason is the preferred drug in a dose of 1 g (two tablets) 4-hourly. Aspirin in high dosage (4–6 g/day) has significant anti-inflammatory as well as analgesic activity, and may therefore achieve a better response than paracetamol in bone pain. Greater flexibility and better tolerance may however be achieved by combining paracetamol with one of the newer non-steroidal anti-inflammatory drugs and this approach is to be preferred in most patients. Proprietary compound tablets have no advantages over either paracetamol or aspirin alone.

Moderate pain. Pain that is unresponsive to simple analgesics is an indication for use of a weak opioid drug. Dextropropoxyphene or dihydrocodeine are the two drugs recommended in this group. Dextropropoxyphene is available as a combination tablet containing dextropropoxyphene 32.5 mg and paracetamol 325 mg (coproxamol) and is recommended in preference to dihydrocodeine because it is theoretically less likely to produce dose-related opioid side-effects, particularly constipation. Whilst dextropropoxyphene has been shown to be an effective analgesic in single doses (Beaver, 1984) there is little evidence from controlled trials that the combination with paracetamol is better than paracetamol alone. When given regularly, however, dose-dependent first pass metabolism and accumulation of its active metabolite norpropoxyphene provide an explanation for the greater clinical efficacy of dextropropoxyphene in both rheumatology (Owen and Hills, 1980) and cancer patients (Hanks and Hoskin, 1986). The usual dose is two tablets of coproxamol 4-hourly, which is in general well-tolerated, though confusion, dysphoria and lightheadedness may occur (particularly in the elderly) and less frequently nausea, vomiting and constipation may become a problem.

Dihydrocodeine given in a dose of 30–60 mg 4-hourly may be used as an alternative but may be accompanied by more prominent opioid side-effects.

Other opioid drugs of similar analgesic strength, including meptazinol, nalbuphine and pentazocine have no particular advantages for use in this situation. Nalbuphine can only be given by injection, meptazinol has a narrow effective dose range with no advantages over coproxamol, and pentazocine is associated with a high incidence of psychotomimetic effects (Hanks and Hoskin, 1987).

Severe pain. For pain that is unresponsive to regular medication with weak opioids, a strong opioid analgesic is required. Morphine is the drug of choice for oral use in this situation, initially in an aqueous formulation given regularly at 4-hourly intervals, and progressing to twice daily controlled-release morphine. A wide dose range is used in patients with advanced cancer, varying from 5 mg to over 1 g 4-hourly. The dose should be titrated against the patient's pain, initiating therapy with 5–10 mg 4-hourly, with no fixed arbitrary upper limit. It is, however, important to note that two-thirds of patients will require no more than 30 mg 4-hourly (Hanks and Twycross, 1984), and careful reassessment to confirm that the pain is morphine-responsive is recommended before escalating the dose beyond these levels. As dose adjustments are made, side-effects may occur and should be anticipated and prevented. Only rarely will true morphine intolerance be encountered provided that active measures are taken to deal with intrusive side-effects. Thus all patients should receive a laxative regularly to avoid constipation, and anti-emetic cover should be provided or made immediately available for the 50–70% of patients who will have associated nausea or vomiting. Drowsiness with poor concentration is a frequent problem on initiating treatment but often resolves spontaneously over a period of a few days so that simple reassurance is usually sufficient.

Respiratory depression does not occur in cancer patients who are receiving oral morphine for pain control, as pain acts as a physiological antagonist to the respiratory effects of opioids (Hanks and Twycross, 1984). Similarly there is no danger of true addiction occurring in these patients despite fears to the contrary. The physical effects of chronic opioid exposure are tolerance (increasing doses of a drug are required to produce the same effect) and physical dependence (physical symptoms of withdrawal ensue if the drug is stopped abruptly). Whilst both tolerance and physical dependence may develop in cancer patients on morphine for periods of weeks or months, the third component of addiction (psychological dependence) is not seen. Psychological dependence accounts for the craving and drug-seeking behaviour seen in addicts, together with their high tendency to relapse back to their addict behaviour patterns when the drug is withdrawn.

The treatment of bone metastases provides a good example of a situation in patients with advanced cancer in which morphine may be used initially to control pain and subsequently be reduced and even discontinued following definitive treatment such as radiotherapy to the site of bone pain. This is illustrated in Figure 2.

There are two formulations of morphine generally available for oral use:

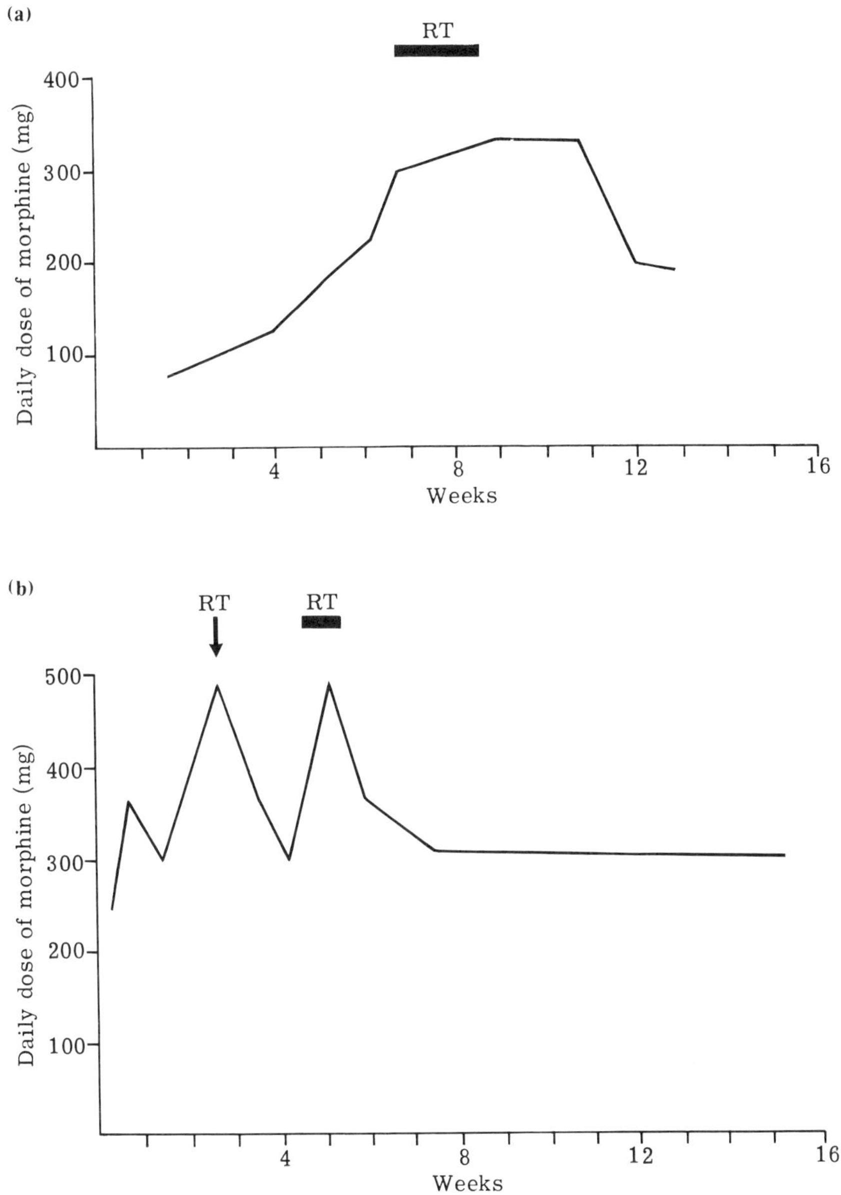

Figure 2. Influence of radiotherapy for local bone pain on morphine requirements. (a) A 61-year-old man with bone metastases from carcinoma of the prostate, who received 30 Gy in 10 daily fractions to the left hip for localized bone pain. (b) A 62-year-old woman with bone metastases from carcinoma of the breast. A single fraction of 8 Gy was given to the right posterior ribs for localized bone pain with good effect. Shortly after this she developed further bone pain in the cervical spine for which she received 20 Gy in five daily fractions. RT = radiotherapy.

morphine elixir, either as a simple aqueous solution or with the addition of a preservative such as chloroform water, and controlled-release morphine tablets (MST-Continus). Whilst the latter provide an ideal means of taking oral morphine when dose requirements are stable, their slow release formulation, resulting in peak concentrations at up to 4-hours after administration (Hanks et al, 1981), makes them unsuitable for patients who are starting treatment with morphine or whose pain is unstable. In these patients dose titration with oral elixir will provide the most rapid pain control and may then be followed by conversion to controlled-release tablets. Bioavailability of morphine from MST is the same as 4-hourly elixir in chronic use in cancer patients (Poulain et al, 1987) and the 12-hourly dose of MST should therefore be the same as the 12-hourly requirement with elixir.

Alternatives to oral morphine will only rarely be required in the treatment of bone pain. If the patient is unable to take oral medication, morphine suppositories are available for rectal use and should be used 4-hourly in the same dose as oral elixir. Oxycodone suppositories are a useful alternative where the rectal route is to be used since they need to be given only 6- to 8-hourly—a 30 mg oxycodone suppository being equivalent to 20 mg oral or rectal morphine.

Where the rectal route is impracticable or unacceptable to the patient, then parenteral medication may be necessary. The subcutaneous route is preferable to intramuscular or intravenous injections, and where parenteral medication is likely to be required for more than 24 hours a continuous infusion using a syringe driver is most appropriate. It is however important to note that injections of strong opioid drugs are not intrinsically more effective in controlling pain than oral medication, and merely provide an alternative means of delivering the drug to opioid receptors in the central nervous system. However, because the drug is well absorbed directly into the systemic circulation, avoiding the extensive first pass metabolism which occurs after oral administration, smaller doses of the drug will be required parenterally. Whilst morphine may be given by this route it has limited solubility in water, the maximum concentration available for injection being 30 mg/ml. Because of this, diamorphine is preferred for parenteral use, being far more soluble with concentrations of up to 250 mg/ml recommended for clinical use (Jones et al, 1985). Whilst there remains controversy over the equivalent doses of oral diamorphine and oral morphine, and of oral versus parenteral morphine or diamorphine during chronic administration, in practice dividing the oral dose of morphine by three will give an appropriate parenteral dose of diamorphine (Hanks and Hoskin, 1987). When given orally, diamorphine has no advantages over morphine, since there is extensive pre-systemic metabolism in the liver, resulting in complete deacetylation of diacetylmorphine to morphine. Following an oral dose of diamorphine, therefore, only morphine can be detected in the systemic circulation (Inturissi et al, 1984).

There are a number of other strong opioid drugs available, none of which have any particular advantage over morphine in the treatment of advanced cancer pain. Potential problems exist in patients who have been receiving these drugs and require a change to morphine since there is a wide range of equivalent doses which it is important to consider before choosing the appropriate starting dose of morphine. Estimations of these doses together with the principal drawbacks of these drugs are shown in Table 1. Where an alternative oral drug is required then phenazocine is recommended, a 5 mg tablet being equivalent to 25 mg morphine taken 4-hourly.

Table 1. Alternative opioids.

Drug	Usual dose (4-hourly unless stated)	Equivalent 4-hourly dose morphine	Disadvantage compared with morphine
Buprenorphine (Temgesic)	0.2 mg 8-hourly	10 mg	Partial agonist Ceiling effect for analgesia
Dextromoramide (Palfium)	5 mg	10 mg	In chronic use short duration of action (1–2 h) and increasing dose requirements
Dipipanone (Diconal, with cyclizine)	10 mg	5 mg	Only available in combination with cyclizine hydrochloride (Diconal)
Nepenthe	10 ml of 10% solution	12 mg	Alcoholic tincture of morphine Variable concentrations available are confusing
Papaveretum (Omnopon)	10 mg	5 mg	Opium extract—active component is morphine
Pethidine	50 mg	6 mg	Short duration of action (2–3 h) In chronic use metabolite toxic to CNS may accumulate causing excitability, tremor, fits
Methadone	5 mg 8-hourly	5 mg	Long half-life, high protein binding. May accumulate with prolonged action, especially in elderly

Co-analgesics

A number of drugs which do not have intrinsic analgesic activity when tested against conventional pain models, may be useful in controlling pain due to advanced cancer when used with one of the analgesic drugs discussed above. Drugs used in this way are co-analgesics (Twycross and Hanks, 1984) and include a wide range of substances such as diuretics, steroids, anticonvulsants, antidepressants and muscle relaxants. They will only be effective where there are specific indications for their use and so careful assessment of the patient's pain and its underlying cause is essential for their correct use.

In the treatment of bone pain, one of the most useful groups of drugs are the non-steroidal anti-inflammatory drugs (NSAIDs). In considering the pathology of bone metastases the possible role for prostaglandins, both in facilitating bone destruction and tumour invasion through activation of osteoclasts, and in modifying neuronal transmission in pain fibres, was discussed. NSAIDs inhibit the synthetic pathway by which arachidonic acid is converted to prostaglandins and this is thought to be their principal mode of action. As primary therapeutic agents NSAIDs are not particularly effective in the treatment of bone metastases and relieve pain in only some 20% of patients (Coombes et al, 1979). However, they may produce worthwhile results when used in conjunction with an opioid analgesic in patients with metastatic bone pain. There is no convincing evidence that any particular NSAID is more efficacious than another in this group of patients. Soluble aspirin is as effective as the newer drugs but its anti-inflammatory action is only seen in high doses of 3.6 g per day or more, and at this level its use may be associated with a significant incidence of side-effects, in particular dyspepsia and gastro-intestinal bleeding. Indomethacin is similarly associated with a high incidence of side-effects but does have the advantage that it can be given by twice daily suppository. For oral use the newer propionic acid derivatives such as ibuprofen, naprosyn or flurbiprofen are generally better tolerated; when a liquid preparation is desirable or where gastric intolerance is a potential problem, benorylate, which is a lipid soluble ester of acetylsalicylic acid and paracetamol, is valuable. This has the additional advantage of needing only twice daily administration in a dose of 5–10 ml (2–4 g).

Since these drugs are potentially hazardous, it is important to carefully assess the patient's response to them without, wherever possible, introducing other variables such as changes in analgesic, and to discontinue the drug where it is clearly ineffective. Particular care is required in the elderly and those with a history of dyspepsia. All the NSAIDs are highly protein-bound and therefore may interact with other protein-bound drugs such as anticoagulants. Care is also needed in patients requiring loop diuretics since many NSAIDs will inhibit their diuretic action (L'Orme, 1986).

In addition to NSAIDs, other co-analgesic drugs may have a role in treating bone pain, particularly where nerve irritation or compression and muscle spasm are present. Corticosteroids are particularly valuable where there is nerve root compression, as they reduce associated oedema and inflammation. Dexamethasone is preferred in this setting in divided doses of 8–16 mg per day, since it is associated with less mineralocorticoid activity which causes the oedema and weight gain seen with steroid treatment. It can also be given in fewer tablets.

Anticonvulsants may be indicated where nerve root irritation is resulting in lancinating or stabbing dysaesthesia or paraesthesia. No particular anticonvulsant drug is superior in this indication and choice is based on individual response and tolerance. In general, clonazepam will be associated with more sedative side-effects than sodium valproate or carbamazepine, but these may cause more gastric irritation. Where muscle spasm is present a muscle relaxant such as baclofen or diazepam may be helpful.

There are anecdotal reports of L-dopa (levodopa) being effective in controlling bone pain due to advanced cancer (Nixon, 1975; Minton et al, 1976) but the only systematic study which has been reported failed to find any evidence of an analgesic effect of L-dopa (used in combination with carbidopa) (Sjolin and Trykker, 1985).

Calcitonin has recently been promoted as effective treatment for bone pain and evidence from case reports and one small prospective randomized study (Hindley et al, 1982) suggests that up to 40% of selected patients can receive useful pain relief following treatment with salmon calcitonin. The main disadvantage of this treatment is the need for multiple subcutaneous injections and the possibility of associated nausea and vomiting, for which anti-emetic cover should be considered. Whilst calcitonin cannot be considered for first line treatment of metastatic bone pain, it may be worth trying where pain persists despite local radiotherapy and appropriate analgesic and co-analgesic therapy.

Mithramycin in relatively low doses (15 mg/kg by weekly intravenous infusion) has been reported to successfully relieve bone pain in metastatic breast cancer (Davies et al, 1979) but no prospective randomized studies confirming this are available.

Radiotherapy

Ionizing radiation is well established in the management of bone pain.

Local external beam irradiation is the treatment of choice for localized metastatic bone pain. The pooled data from 16 non-randomized reports of treating patients in this way using a wide range of radiation doses reveals that in a total of 2422 treatments a mean overall response rate of 86% (range 73–100) and mean *complete* response rate of 52% (range 20–90) is found (Hoskin, 1988). No evidence for a dose–response relationship is seen nor any advantage for prolonged multiple fraction therapy. There is no clear difference in response between various types of primary tumour, and, although many patients in these series have only limited survival, response in terms of pain relief is prolonged, being maintained in 78% of patients at five years from treatment in one series (Allen et al, 1976). Many criticisms can however be made of these data in which little detail is given of treatment techniques, criteria for diagnosis, dose definition and correction, or patient selection where more than one dose fractionation schedule has been used. Only four of these 16 reports have employed prospective pain assessments, the remainder using a retrospective assessment of case records, and all use physician rather than patient assessment, which will tend to overestimate response rates.

There are three prospective randomized trials of radiotherapy in metastatic bone pain (Tong et al, 1982; Madsen, 1983; Price et al, 1986a). The results from these trials support the retrospective and non-randomized data with overall response rates of 90%, 48% and 85% respectively. In these three studies, a range of radiation doses have been randomly allocated, including a single fraction of 8 Gy, two fractions of 10 Gy in one week, six fractions of 4 Gy in three weeks and 15 fractions of 2.7 Gy in three weeks. No consistent advantage for any one particular dose fractionation schedule emerges from these three studies, although a re-analysis of the earliest trial has suggested an advantage for multiple fractions (Blitzer, 1985). Duration of response has also been investigated in these studies and overall about one half of patients have response lasting until death. In those surviving up to one year from treatment 60% were still responding with no significant differential effect of radiation dose or fractionation being seen. Long-term survivors tend to have primary tumours of breast or prostate and Tong et al have suggested that these tumours show better response than other histological types. This is not confirmed in other studies where no difference between histological groups is seen.

There is then little doubt that external beam radiotherapy is a highly effective treatment for localized bone pain due to tumour metastases, where response rates of some 80% can be anticipated. Since a single fraction treatment appears as effective as multiple fractions this will be the preferred means of delivery for most patients where pain relief is the primary aim of treatment. Where irradiation is being performed for prophylaxis of, or stabilization of, pathological fractures then many radiotherapists will prefer to use a fractionated regimen, delivering 30 Gy in 10 daily fractions or its equivalent. Similarly, fractionated regimens are often preferred for large fields such as the pelvis or certain histological types of tumour thought to be relatively radioresistant, such as renal carcinoma, although there are few data to support this approach.

Whilst external beam therapy offers the optimal treatment for localized bone pain, unfortunately most bone metastases arising from blood-borne spread of tumour emboli are multiple, and frequently the patient will have several sites of pain. Isolated treatment of one site in these patients will often serve only to unmask pain in another site which will then require further treatment, and so the cycle will be repeated. In this situation, wide field irradiation, in which the upper, middle or lower hemi-body is encompassed in a single radiation volume, may be appropriate. A review of five reported series in the literature (Hoskin, 1988) shows that single fraction hemi-body irradiation delivering 6–8 Gy mid-plane dose will produce a response in about 75% of patients. Response is often rapid (within 24–48 hours), with a duration of several months or until death. Against this must be balanced the greater toxicity of wide-field irradiation. Virtually all patients suffer mild gastro-intestinal toxicity with nausea and diarrhoea within the first 48 hours after treatment. Bone marrow depression is seen in some 10% of patients unless sequential upper and lower hemi-body irradiation is performed, when most patients will have significant falls in blood count. Pneumonitis from upper hemi-body irradiation in this setting has been reported in 10% or more of patients (Fitzpatrick, 1981; Qasim, 1981) and subsequent treatment-related deaths may be seen from this complication. Toxicity may be minimized by careful preparation, premedication with steroids, anti-emetics and sedatives, and regular monitoring of the blood count with haematological support and treatment of infections in neutropenic patients. Pneumonitis is a dose-related complication and is rare when doses to the upper hemi-body are limited to 6 Gy uncorrected for lung density.

Careful patient selection is therefore necessary for this procedure but in suitable patients with widespread bone metastases, particularly those from myeloma or carcinoma of the prostate, wide field irradiation delivering 6 Gy mid-plane dose to the upper hemi-body or 8 Gy mid-plane dose to the lower hemi-body will provide useful pain relief in some 75% of patients. Isolated painful areas that persist or arise due to subsequent disease progression may still be treated by local radiotherapy if necessary without additional problems (Epstein et al, 1979).

An alternative approach to the treatment of multiple bone pain from scattered metastases has been the systemic administration of radioisotopes selectively taken up by bone. Early studies with radioactive phosphorus (^{32}P) showed that this method of treatment could be effective in selected patients, but when doses of up to 21 mCi of ^{32}P were given over six weeks, bone marrow suppression was found in most patients (Tong, 1971). More recent work has focused on the use of strontium (^{87}Sr) which is preferentially concentrated and retained in areas of osteoblastic activity but delivers a lower overall dose to the bone marrow (Robinson, 1986). Response rates varying from 51–86% are reported in the literature in selected groups of patients (Hoskin, 1988) with little or no bone marrow suppression, and subsequent treatment to localized sites with external beam radiotherapy was not compromised. This is clearly an area for further research, requiring prospective randomized studies to define the role of such radioisotopes in the management of widespread bone pain and also to explore newer techniques of localization such as the use of labelled diphosphonates.

Surgery

The role of surgery in the management of bone pain due to metastatic cancer is limited but may be invaluable where there is impending pathological fracture or a displaced unstable fracture through a metastatic deposit. Lytic deposits in a weight-bearing long bone carry a high risk of subsequent fracture once there is erosion of cortical bone. Spontaneous healing of such fractures is unlikely despite adequate immobilization. Left untreated the patient will experience severe pain on movement and usually succumb from the consequent immobilization. In these cases internal fixation using an intramedullary nail or prosthetic replacement of the upper femur will stabilize the fracture, enable good pain relief to be achieved and usually allow the patient to become mobile once more.

Chemotherapy and hormone therapy

Since the underlying cause for bone pain due to metastatic cancer is the growing malignant tumour, the most rational response to this is to give treatment which will result in tumour shrinkage and control of its subsequent growth and further spread. Unfortunately, in the population of patients presenting with bone pain, two thirds will have primary tumours such as lung, prostate, or kidney for which no effective chemotherapeutic agents are available (Price et al, 1986a). Therefore chemotherapy will only be appropriate in a minority of patients, predominantly those with breast cancer or myeloma, and in this group treatment with appropriate chemotherapy regimens should be considered for widespread bone pain, particularly if there is active disease elsewhere. In carcinoma of the breast, which may account for up to one third of patients presenting with bone pain (Price et al, 1986a), chemotherapy will be considered for those patients who have failed to respond to hormone therapy or who are pre-menopausal with oestrogen receptor negative tumours, or those with aggressive widespread disease. Depending upon the drug regimen used, complete response rates for bone metastases ranging from 0 to 84% are reported. A rapid response in terms of pain relief is unusual, the median time to achieve maximal response in bone metastases being 32 weeks, which is considerably longer than in other tissues (Whitehouse, 1985).

The high relative incidence of carcinoma of the breast and prostate amongst patients presenting with bone pain, both of which are hormone sensitive tumours, means that therapy utilizing a form of endocrine manipulation may be considered in these patients. Pain relief may be rapid, within 24 hours of an ablative hormone manoeuvre, and frequently occurs despite no objective changes in either bone or soft tissue tumours (Stoll, 1985). A 'pain flare' may also be seen on initiating or changing hormone therapy, as may hypercalcaemia, but despite this about one half of patients experiencing such a 'flare' will subsequently go on to achieve pain relief. In breast cancer a number of therapeutic options are available, all of which may be effective in bone pain. With older treatments such as oestrogen, androgen or steroid therapy, response rates for bone pain of approximately 25% are found, and a slightly higher response rate of 35% is reported with ablative procedures such as oophorectomy, adrenalectomy or hypophysectomy. Today, hormone manipulation is usually achieved using either tamoxifen, aminoglutethimide or a progestogen. With both tamoxifen and progestogens response rates for bone pain in the region of 20% are reported, but aminoglutethimide given with hydrocortisone, when compared with tamoxifen as first-line therapy in prospective randomized studies, appears to have a consistently higher response rate in bone of about 35% (Smith and Macaulay, 1985).

In carcinoma of the prostate, orchiectomy is the hormone treatment of first choice today, having similar response rates but none of the cardiovascular complications of oestrogen therapy. Some 85% of patients will respond to their first-line endocrine manoeuvre. Subsequent relapse is however more difficult to manage using systemic therapy. Response rates to a second hormone manoeuvre such as stilboestrol, cyproterone acetate or luteinizing hormone releasing hormone (LHRH) analogues are poor. Aminoglutethimide with hydrocortisone has been reported to produce response in about one third of patients when used as a second-line agent (Catalona, 1984), and may be the endocrine treatment of choice for patients with prostatic cancer relapsing after orchiectomy with bone pain, although a recent study has suggested that hydrocortisone alone may produce similar response rates (Plowman et al, 1987). At present 4-hydroxyandrostenedione is under investigation for the treatment of bone pain in advanced prostatic cancer; early results are encouraging (Shearer R.J., 1987, personal communication) but further studies with this agent are required before more widespread use can be recommended.

In addition to these hormone-dependent tumours, relief from bone pain has been reported following hypophysectomy in tumours not generally

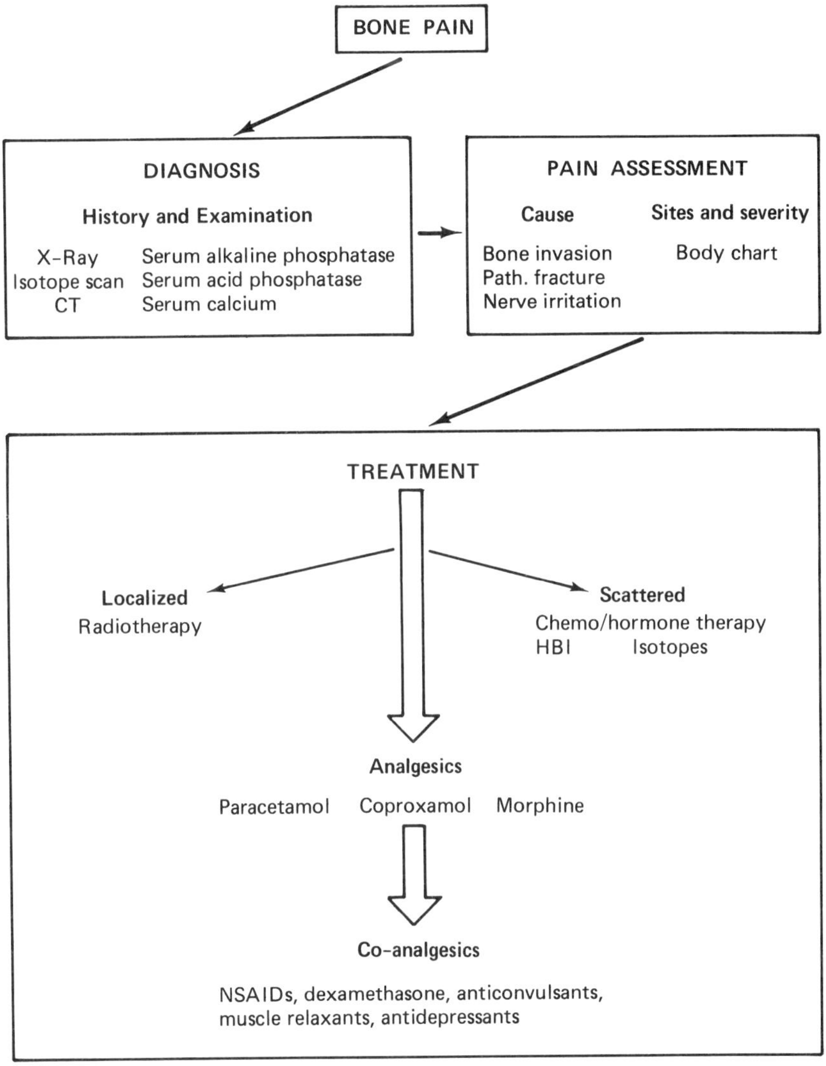

Figure 3. Summary of management of bone pain. HBI = hemi-body irradiation.

recognized to be hormone sensitive. It is unclear whether this represents a true endocrine response or is due to other sequelae of hypophysectomy such as damage to pain fibres in the vicinity, changes in endogenous endorphins, or the need for hormone supplements such as cortisone (Stoll, 1985). Such manoeuvres are, however, unlikely to form a routine part in the management of bone pain.

CONCLUSION

Bone pain from metastatic disease is a common problem in patients with advanced cancer. Effective treatment is available for the majority of patients based on careful diagnosis and assessment of the pain, and the application of a simple analgesic ladder supplemented by the use of appropriate co-analgesic drugs, radiotherapy, surgery, chemotherapy or hormone therapy, as summarized in Figure 3.

Acknowledgement

We are extremely grateful to Mrs F. Fleetwood for typing the manuscript. PJ Hoskin is supported by the Cancer Research Campaign.

REFERENCES

Abrams HL, Spiro R & Goldstein N (1950) Metastases in carcinoma: analysis of 1000 autopsied cases. *Cancer* **3:** 74–85.

Allen KL, Johnson TW & Hibbs GG (1976) Effective bone palliation as related to various treatment regimes. *Cancer* **37:** 984–986.

Beaver WT (1984) Analgesic efficacy of dextropropoxyphene and dextropropoxyphene-containing combinations: a review. *Human Toxicology* **3:** 1915–2205.

Blitzer PH (1985) Reanalysis of the RTOG study of the palliation of symptomatic osseous metastasis. *Cancer* **55:** 1468–1472.

Carter R (1985) Patterns and mechanisms of localized bone invasion by tumors: studies with squamous carcinoma of the head and neck. *CRC Critical Reviews in Clinical Laboratory Sciences* **22:** 275–315.

Catalona WJ (1984) Endocrine Therapy. In *Prostate Cancer*, pp 145–172. Orlando: Grune and Stratton.

Coombes RC, Munro Neville A, Gazet J-C et al (1979) Agents affecting osteolysis in patients with breast cancer. *Cancer Chemotherapy and Pharmacology* **3:** 41–44.

Cranston PE, Patel RB & Harrison RB (1984) Computed tomography for metastatic lesions of the osseous pelvis. *Journal of Computer Assisted Tomography* **8:** 582.

Davies J, Trask C & Souhami RL (1979) Effect of mithramycin on widespread painful bone metastases from cancer of the breast. *Cancer Treatment Reports* **63:** 1835–1838.

Edelstyn GA, Gillespie PJ & Grebbell FS (1967) The radiological demonstration of osseous metastases: experimental observations. *Clinical Radiology* **18:** 158–162.

Epstein LM, Stewart BH, Antunez AR et al (1979) Half and total body radiation for carcinoma of the prostate. *Journal of Urology* **122:** 330–332.

Ferreira SH (1972) Prostaglandins, aspirin-like drugs and analgesia. *Nature* (New Biology) **240:** 200–203.

Fitzpatrick PJ (1981) Wide-field irradiation of bone metastases. In Weiss L & Gilbert HA (eds) *Bone Metastases*, pp 399–427. Boston: G.K. Hall.

Galasko CSB (1981) The development of skeletal metastases. In Weiss L & Gilbert HA (eds) *Bone Metastases*, pp 83–113. Boston: G.K. Hall.

Goris ML & Bretille J (1985) Skeletal scintigraphy for the diagnosis of malignant metastatic disease to the bones. *Radiotherapy and Oncology* **3:** 319–329.

Hanks GW (1983) Adverse effects of acetylsalicyl acid. *Clinical Therapeutics* **5**(supplement B): 5–8.

Hanks GW & Hoskin PJ (1986) Pain control in advanced cancer: pharmacological methods. *Journal of the Royal College of Physicians of London* **20:** 276–281.

Hanks GW & Hoskin PJ (1987) Opioid analgesics. *Palliative Medicine* **1:** 1–25.

Hanks GW & Twycross RG (1984) Pain, the physiological antagonist of opioid analgesics. *Lancet* **i:** 1477–1478.

Hanks GW, Rose NM, Aherne GW et al (1981) Controlled release morphine tablets: a double blind trial in dental surgery patients. *British Journal of Anaesthesia* **53:** 1259–1264.
Hindley AC, Hill AB, Leyland MJ & Wiles AE (1982) A double-blind controlled trial of salmon calcitonin in pain due to malignancy. *Cancer Chemotherapy and Pharmacology* **9:** 71–74.
Horton EW (1963) Action of prostaglandin E_1 on tissues which respond to bradykinin. *Nature* **200:** 892–893.
Hoskin PJ (1988) Scientific and clinical aspects of radiotherapy in the relief of bone pain. *Cancer Surveys* **7:** (in press).
Inturissi CE, Max MB, Foley KM et al (1984) The pharmacokinetics of heroin in patients with chronic pain. *New England Journal of Medicine* **310:** 1213–1217.
Jacobs SC (1983) Spread of prostatic cancer to bone. *Urology* **21:** 337–344.
Jones V, Murphy A & Hanks GW (1985) Stability of diamorphine. *Pharmaceutical Journal* **235:** 426.
L'Orme ME (1986) Non-steroidal antiinflammatory drugs and the kidney. *British Medical Journal* **292:** 1621–1622.
Madsen EL (1983) Painful bone metastasis: efficacy of radiotherapy assessed by the patients: a randomized trial comparing 4 Gy × 6 versus 10 Gy × 2. *International Journal of Radiation Oncology, Biology, Physics* **9:** 1775–1779.
Minton JP, Bronn DG & Kibbey WE (1976) L-Dopa effect in painful bony metastases. *New England Journal of Medicine* **294:** 340.
Nixon DW (1975) Use of L-Dopa to relieve pain from bone metastases. *New England Journal of Medicine* **292:** 647.
Owen M & Hills LJ (1980) How safe is dextropropoxyphene? *Medical Journal of Australia* **1:** 617.
Plowman PN, Perry LA & Chard T (1987) Androgen suppression by hydrocortisone without aminoglutethimide in orchiectomised men with prostatic cancer. *British Journal of Urology* **59:** 255–257.
Poulain P, Hanks GW, Walker VA, Aherne GW, Hoskin PJ & Littleton P (1987) The relative bioavailability of controlled release morphine tablets in cancer patients I: serum morphine measured by RIA (in press).
Powles TJ, Dowsett M, Easty DM, Easty GC & Neville AM (1976) Breast cancer osteolysis, bone metastases and anti-osteolytic effect of aspirin. *Lancet* **i:** 608–610.
Price P, Hoskin PJ, Easton D et al (1986a) Prospective randomised trial of single and multi-fraction radiotherapy schedules in the treatment of painful bony metastases. *Radiotherapy and Oncology* **6:** 247–255.
Price P, Hoskin PJ, Easton D et al (1986b) Optimal dose and fractionation of radiotherapy required to palliate painful bone metastases (Abstract). *Proceedings of the British Oncological Association*, 1986.
Qasim MM (1981) Half body irradiation (HBI) in metastatic carcinomas. *Clinical Radiology* **32:** 215–219.
Rainsbury RM, Ott RJ, Westwood JH et al (1983) Localisation of metastatic breast carcinoma by a monoclonal antibody labelled with Indium-III. *Lancet* **ii:** 934–938.
Rimmer WD, Berquist TH, McLeod RA et al (1985) Bone tumours: magnetic resonance imaging versus computed tomography. *Radiology* **155:** 709–718.
Robinson RG (1986) Radionuclides for the alleviation of bone pain in advanced malignancy. *Clinics in Oncology* **5:** 39–49.
Sheedy RA, McLeod DH, Stephens DH, Hattery RR & Beabout JW (1977) CT and the musculoskeletal system. *Journal of Computer Assisted Tomography* **1:** 362.
Sjolin SU & Trykker H (1985) Unsuccessful treatment of severe pain from bone metastases with Sinemet 25/100. *New England Journal of Medicine* **312:** 650–651.
Smith IE & Macaulay V (1985) Comparison of different endocrine therapies in management of bone metastases from breast carcinoma. *Journal of the Royal Society of Medicine* **78** (supplement 9): 15–21.
Stoll BA (1985) Mechanisms in endocrine therapy of bone metastases. *Journal of the Royal Society of Medicine* **78** (supplement 9): 11–14.
Tong ECK (1971) Parathormone and ^{32}P therapy in prostatic cancer with bone metastases. *Radiology* **98:** 343–351.

Tong D, Gillick L & Hendrickson FR (1982) The palliation of symptomatic osseous metastases: final results of the study by the Radiation Therapy Oncology Group. *Cancer* **50:** 893–899.
Twycross RG & Fairfield S (1982) Pain in far advanced cancer. *Pain* **14:** 303–310.
Twycross RG & Hanks GW (1984) Coanalgesia. *Clinics in Oncology* **3:** 153–164.
Whitehouse JMA (1985) Site-dependant response to chemotherapy for carcinoma of the breast. *Journal of the Royal Society of Medicine* **78** (supplement 9): 18–22.

10

Recent advances in the control of pain

MATTHEW E. CONOLLY

'For all the happiness Mankind can gain
Is not in pleasure but in rest from pain.'
(*The Indian Emperour*, Act IV, Scene i,
John Dryden. 1667)

Three million patients dying from cancer each year experience significant pain, as do 16 million of those with less advanced cancer. Numerous studies suggest that at least a half of this prodigious number are never adequately treated (Bonica, 1985). This sombre observation compels us to examine the effectiveness with which we use the knowledge we already have, and gives great urgency to the quest for therapeutic innovations to provide 'rest from pain'.

The perception of pain

Historically the relief of pain has advanced backwards, insofar as morphine (known for 3000 years) and the non-steroidal anti-inflammatory drugs (as represented by aspirin, which was introduced in the nineteenth century) were used to alleviate pain long before there was any understanding of how pain was perceived, or how these drugs were able to modify the process.

In recent years, neurophysiological and histochemical studies have begun to unravel the complexities of the pathways whereby nociceptive impulses from the periphery are relayed centrally, and then either suppressed, or else transmitted rostrally, ultimately to be perceived as pain. From such studies, new approaches to the control of pain must ultimately emerge.

Sensory receptors (nociceptors) that are preferentially responsive to tissue damaging stimuli are found in the skin, muscles, joints, connective tissue and abdominal and thoracic viscera. Most studies involving nociceptors and their response to stimuli have, for obvious reasons, focussed on superficial structures. However the mechanisms operating in deeper tissues, from which most cancer-related pain comes, may not be the same (Wall, 1985).

Nociceptors appear to be of two types, myelinated and non-myelinated. The myelinated ones relay signals to the spinal cord via the lightly myelinated Aδ fibres which have a conduction velocity of 5–50 m/s. They respond preferentially (albeit not exclusively) to mechanical stimuli, to which they are far more responsive than are the non-myelinated type. Non-myelinated nociceptors respond to a wider range of stimuli (mechanical, thermal and chemical), and relay signals via the slower (non-myelinated) c fibres.

A number of compounds have been thought to sensitize nociceptors. In malignant disease especially it seems likely that such a mechanism could be important, since the level of pain experienced by the patient is not always commensurate with the demonstrable degree of tissue damage. Conversely, pain (from a bony metastasis for example) may be relieved long before a fully effective dose of radiotherapy has been delivered. Compounds proposed for this sensitizing role have included acetylcholine, histamine, 5-hydroxytryptamine, H^+ and K^+ ions, prostaglandins E_1 and E_2, leukotrienes, bradykinin and substance P. There are data to suggest that each of these acting alone (Chahl 1979), or more than one acting in concert (Taira and Nakano, 1974) may act in this way, although none have been unequivocally established in this role, and there remains the tantalizing possibility that other compounds capable of sensitizing nociceptors remain to be discovered.

It has become increasingly clear that the spinal cord is far from being a passive conduit for pain signals arriving from the periphery. The dorsal horn, wherein the neurons entering the cord form synapses with ascending neurons, is an area of great complexity. Aδ fibres form synapses in the most superficial layer of the dorsal horn (lamina I) and part of lamina II and III, while the unmyelinated c fibres mostly terminate at synapses in lamina II. The cells whose dendrites form the 'central' part of these synapses decussate and ascend as the neospinothalamic and paleospinothalamic tracts. Fibres of the neospinothalamic tract form synapses in the ventrobasilar thalamic complex, whence axons project to the parietal cortex. In contrast, axons of the paleospinothalamic tract form synapses with cells of the reticular formation of the brain-stem, the posterior thalamic nucleus, and the central lateral nucleus of the intralaminar thalamic nuclear complex. From these thalamic synapses, projections to many cortical areas arise. The ultimate projections of the neospinothalamic tract are thought to be concerned with discriminative aspects of pain perception (localization and intensity), while those of the paleospinothalamic system are more concerned with the emotional and affective components of pain (Payne, 1987).

Before an impulse can pass from the axon entering the dorsal horn and ascend to higher centres, it is subject to the modulating influence of a variety of interneurons and descending fibres, the details of which are not yet completely understood (Basbaum, 1985). For the most part these neuronal connections appear to serve an inhibitory function, serving to block the rostral transmission of the nociceptive information. These inhibitory signals may originate from segmental interneurons which utilize enkephalins, dynorphin or γ-aminobutyric acid (GABA) as their neurotransmitter. Another major inhibitory mechanism is vested in the descending bulbospinal tract. These neurons appear to be noradrenergic or serotonergic. Whether they inhibit by a direct action on the spinothalamic tract, or by an indirect action via the above-mentioned interneurons has not yet been determined. This imprecise understanding is the underpinning of the 'gate' mechanism of pain control that resulted in the clinical exploitation of transcutaneous electrical nerve stimulation (Wall and Sweet, 1967). It forms the basis of the rationale for the use of epidural and intrathecal opiates as a form of analgesic therapy, and it provides a partial explanation for the somewhat controversial use of adrenergic and serotonergic tricyclic anti-depressants as co-analgesics.

Another aspect of the complexity of spinal cord neurophysiology which is of relevance to the perception of pain is the phenomenon of 'functional plasticity', best exemplified by the studies of Woolf (1983). Using chronically decerebrate rats, he has shown that an acute thermal injury will lead to an exaggerated response to mechanical stimuli, characterized not only by a decreased threshold to mechanical stimuli in the area of the original injury, but also by exaggerated responsiveness in parts *beyond* the area of the original injury. Once induced, these changes may last for several days. Possibly of relevance to the question of cancer pain is the observation that in these animal studies assaults on deep structures produced a far greater degree of excitability in the spinal cord than did cutaneous injuries. It is also noteworthy that although input via a peripheral nerve is necessary to establish such excitability, once it is established it becomes independent of ongoing peripheral input, and blockade of sensory nerves from the injured tissue does not cause a reversion to normal (Woolf, 1985). The nature of the changes underlying this phenomenon is at present quite unknown. It is tempting to speculate that changes in some of the polysynaptic inhibitory mechanisms mentioned above might be involved. Unravelling the neurophysiology of functional plasticity may provide valuable leads to new forms of analgesic therapy for patients with incurable malignancies.

The causes of pain in malignant disease

It is a straightforward enough (though often neglected) observation that patients with malignant disease very often have not one, but several, causes of pain. It may be due to the malignant process itself, it may be a consequence of therapy aimed at the malignancy, or it may be due to some coincidental but strictly unrelated process. As described by Twycross and Lack (1984) 81% of patients with malignant disease have at least two independent causes of pain, while 34% have four or more separate painful conditions. These same authors also point out that the clinical pattern can change quite markedly from day to day, so that not only is a thorough initial investigation needed, but frequent review of each patient is also vital. In light of this, the attempt by some governmental agencies to equate terminal care with denial of access to investigative procedures speaks eloquently of ignorance and insensitivity. Assessment of the patient calls for a careful history, a thorough examination, and the performance of whatever diagnostic tests may be indicated (X-ray, computerized tomography (CT) scan, magnetic resonance imaging *etc.*). Attention must also be paid to the patient's social and psychological state. An important observation of Dame Cicely Saunders is that what the patient experiences, his 'Total Pain', commonly has four components. These she has labelled physical pain, social pain, mental pain and spiritual pain (Saunders, 1984). If the physician focusses all his attention on the alleviation of physical pain, while ignoring the fact that the patient is overwhelmed by, say, mental anguish, it is not likely that he will afford his patient much relief.

Pain caused by the malignant process

Bony involvement. This is the commonest cause of pain in malignant disease (Wall, 1985) although some bony metastases cause no pain. Nociceptors are found in the periosteum and in the joint tissues, but not in the cortex or marrow. Once 25% of the cortex has been eroded, the patient is at risk of developing a pathological fracture. When 75% has been destroyed, such a fracture becomes almost inevitable. However, as noted above, the degree of pain does not always correlate with the extent of actual bony involvement. This prompts the idea of a chemical agent being the originator of the pain. Although prostaglandins have often been implicated in the development of pain arising from metastases, their role is not always clear. Pain is usually well localized, although if the tumour involves adjacent neuronal structures, particularly around the base of the skull, remote symptoms may also arise (Foley, 1987).

Visceral involvement. Invasion of thoracic or abdominal viscera produces a poorly localized pain of a constant aching quality. Excitation of cells of the spinothalamic tract by visceral afferents may render these cells unusually responsive to low intensity signals from the related dermatome, thus providing a basis for the referred pain and tenderness commonly associated with visceral involvement (Pomeranz et al, 1968).

Tumour infiltration of nerves. Neuronal damage causing neuropathic pain is rightly feared. The pain is a constant burning, searing, aching sensation, on which paroxysms of shooting, stabbing or shock-like pains are superimposed. Typically such pain is very resistant to conventional analgesic therapy. It may arise when sensory pathways are interrupted at any point between the periphery and the cerebral cortex, and because it is believed to be related to loss of normal neuronal input, it has come to be referred to as *deafferentation* pain. Sometimes, but not always, when there is a partial nerve lesion there is an accompanying sensory deficit, and commonly an exaggerated and unpleasant perception of a normally harmless stimulus (hyperpathia). The latter disappears once the damaging involvement of the nerve progresses to total denervation.

Distinct clinical pictures involving neuropathic pain emerge according to which nerves are affected.

1. Radicular pain may be felt if nerves are involved in the intercostal, paravertebral or retroperitoneal spaces. Pain extending down the arm is characteristic of involvement of the brachial plexus.

2. The Pancoast syndrome caused by invasion of the plexus from below initially affects the medial aspect of the arm, forearm and hand.
3. Infiltration from breast cancer may initially involve the higher segments of the brachial plexus, though obviously this will be very variable. The onset of such pain may be the first warning of tumour infiltration. Pain may be experienced for weeks or months before objective neurological signs develop.
4. Infiltration of the lumbosacral plexus is potentially the most disruptive because of the combination of pain and loss of mobility caused by paralysis of the legs. CT scan and myelography seem to be the most useful techniques for establishing the diagnosis.
5. Meningeal metastases commonly cause constant pain in the head, neck and/or lower back, and may be difficult to distinguish from arachnoiditis and fungal or other meningitides.

Pain caused by cancer therapy

Some of these pains are not exclusive to patients with cancer. Acute post-operative pain is to be expected, and should be readily controlled.

Surgery which involves extensive dissection and nerve damage may give rise to deafferentation pain of the type described above. Surgery involving the loss of substantial amounts of muscle may give rise to myofascial pain in the remaining muscle. When nerves regenerate after being severed, the sprouting ends may form neuromata. These structures differ from normal neural tissue in that they fire spontaneously, they are sensitive to mechanical stimuli, and they can be excited by α-adrenergic stimulation (Wall, 1985). Typical sites for troublesome neuromata include the intercostal nerves after thoracotomy, the intercostobrachial nerve after mastectomy, and the first lumbar nerve after nephrectomy. In addition, painful neuromata in the stumps of amputated limbs are well known. The late recurrence of phantom limb pain in a limb previously amputated for malignant disease may be an early warning of proximal recurrence (Foley, 1987).

Chemotherapy may also give rise to pain. Cisplatin and the vinca alkaloids (notably vincristine) are common offenders producing burning sensations in the hands and feet. Pain may also complicate steroid therapy (aseptic necrosis of bone), and non-steroidal anti-inflammatory drug therapy (peptic ulceration).

Radiotherapy also may give rise to pain. Acutely an irradiated breast may be painful and this can last for several weeks or months. Chronically radiation-induced fibrosis may involve and damage nerves, giving rise to painful situations sometimes many years after the event, making the distinction between radiation and recurrence a difficult diagnostic problem. Involvement of the brachial plexus in patients with breast cancer may lead to a painful and paralysed limb. Damage to the spinal cord producing a myelopathy, characterized by pain and the development of a Brown-Séquard syndrome may sometimes be seen.

NEW APPROACHES TO THE TREATMENT OF CANCER PAIN

For simplicity, acceptability to the patient, and for the sake of universal availability, the development of drugs suitable for *oral* administration must remain at the centre of new therapeutic strategies to deal with cancer pain. This is not to deny the importance of other techniques such as chronic morphine infusions, or some of the more sophisticated neurosurgical techniques, but expense, lack of equipment, and lack of availability of skilled nursing support will put these forever out of reach of most of suffering humanity.

Mild analgesics

These compounds remain the first approach to the management of cancer pain, at least in its early stages. Included in this group are the non-steroidal anti-inflammatory drugs (NSAIDs), paracetamol (acetaminophen), and opiates of low potency.

Aspirin was the first, and remains the best known of the NSAIDs, though recent years have seen the emergence of a multitude of new compounds. Only zomepirac has clearly greater anti-inflammatory effects than aspirin, though drugs such as ibuprofen, sulindac, diclofenac and piroxicam have fewer gastric side-effects. Piroxicam, naproxen and diflunisal have a long duration of action, and so may be given less frequently than aspirin. Paracetamol is comparable to aspirin as an analgesic, though with little anti-inflammatory effect, being relatively inactive against cyclo-oxygenases in the peripheral tissues. Probably for this reason it causes no gastric irritation.

The NSAIDs have a definite ceiling to their analgesic action, so with one important exception are not very useful in controlling cancer pain of high intensity. This exception is relief of pain from bony metastases, where adequate deployment of these drugs is of crucial importance and may, on occasion, allow opiates to be discontinued, at least for a while (Baines and Kirkham, 1984).

The range of applicability of NSAIDs has been extended by combining them with weak opiates (see below) with which they act synergistically. Preparations such as Tylenol/codeine (paracetamol + codeine), Distalgesic (dextropropoxyphene + paracetamol), Percocet (paracetamol + oxycodone) and Percodan (oxycodone + aspirin) are widely used and are considered to be helpful, even though rigorous clinical trials of their efficacy are few.

Opiates

Recent years have seen substantial advances in our knowledge of opiate pharmacology. The discovery of endogenous opiates (enkephalins and endorphins) led to the recognition of the endogenous pain control mechanisms mentioned above. It is now understood that not all opiate receptors are the same, but that there are at least five different sub-types, μ_1, μ_2, δ, κ and σ. Likewise, opiate drugs are not uniform. Some are agonists, exhibiting relative selectivity for one or more receptor. Of these, some are full agonists, while others are partial agonists. Some drugs exert purely antagonistic actions at the opiate receptor, and may be used like naloxone to antagonize the action of morphine. Others more recently developed exert a mixture of agonist and antagonist actions (see Table 1).

Table 1. Method of action of opiates.

	Agonists	Agonist/antagonist
Weak opiates	Codeine Dextropropoxyphene Dihydrocodeine	Pentazocine
Strong opiates	Diamorphine (heroin) Hydromorphone Methadone Morphine Oxycodone Oxymorphone Pethidine (meperidine)	Buprenorphine Butorphanol Nalbuphine

The weak opiates are analgesics of limited usefulness. The ones currently available are codeine, dihydrocodeine (not available in USA), propoxyphene (dextropropoxyphene in UK), and pentazocine. Though limited in their ability to relieve pain, as opiates they exhibit anticipated side-effects such as nausea and constipation. Their abuse potential is minimal. They are generally used in fixed dose combinations with NSAIDs, which makes it impossible to give them in large doses without giving unacceptably large doses of the NSAID at the same time. Oxycodone is often erroneously considered to be a weak opiate analgesic for this very reason.

The development of opiates with both agonist and antagonist properties was motivated by a desire to produce a drug free from some of the undesirable side-effects of morphine such as dependence and respiratory depression. However, at least in the context of cancer, this concern is misplaced. Respiratory depression does not occur if the dose of morphine is titrated carefully against the pain to be relieved (Walsh et al, 1981). Furthermore, even though an agonist/antagonist drug will exert an analgesic (opiate agonist) effect at low to moderate doses, as the dose increases so the antagonist effect becomes more pronounced, and beyond a certain point no further increase in pain relief can be achieved. Even more troublesome if such a drug is given in combination with a pure agonist such as morphine, the net effect is to antagonize the action of morphine. In clinical terms this causes a significant exacerbation of pain and often symptoms of opiate withdrawal. There seems therefore no real place for these agents in the management of cancer pain.

Morphine remains the strong opiate of choice in almost all circumstances. The world owes a great debt to the Hospice movement which has rediscovered knowledge which is centuries old—namely that morphine can perfectly well be given by mouth if the patient has a normal gut. True, only about one third of an oral dose reaches the systemic circulation, but that is of no consequence so long as, when changing from parenteral to oral administration (or vice versa), the appropriate adjustment in dose is made.

Another advance in the proper use of morphine, established by Dr Saunders and her colleagues 20 years ago but still not widely enough known, is that morphine must be given on a *time-contingent* basis, in a dose large enough to *keep* the pain suppressed. It is tragic that this point should have to appear in a review dealing with recent advances, but casual inspection of prescription orders in University teaching hospitals reveals that opiates all too often are still prescribed:

(a) parenterally when it is not necessary to do so;
(b) in inadequate doses;
(c) 'p.r.n. for pain'.

It is clear that in the minds of many physicians recurrent pain is regarded as acceptable. 'Millions of people suffer daily from cancer pain without receiving adequate treatment . . . pain is most poorly managed in those most defenceless against it—the young and the elderly' (Liebeskind and Melzack, 1987). The reasons for this sorry state of affairs is largely misinformation concerning the pharmacology of opiates, which allows the perpetuation of various myths. For example:

'If I give you morphine now it will have lost its effect when we really need it.' The truth is that when opiates are given regularly in an appropriate dose, the dosage requirements remain remarkably stable for a long period of time (Twycross, 1984). Dramatic increases in dose requirement are only likely to be seen in the very terminal phases of the malignancy, when extension of the tumour encroaches on nerves giving rise to neuropathic pain. Although this is sometimes erroneously thought of as tolerance, the abrupt increase in morphine requirement makes it quite clear that 'tolerance' has nothing to do with it (Foley, 1985).

'I don't want to give you morphine in case you become addicted.' This also is a false premise. It has been observed repeatedly that if an alternative pain strategy (such as nerve block or cordotomy) is adopted, opiates can be withdrawn rapidly, with relatively little in the way of withdrawal symptoms. Patients may transiently experience such symptoms but do not exhibit drug-seeking behaviour (Twycross, 1984; Foley, 1985).

Oral morphine

An innovation in the use of oral morphine whose simplicity belies its usefulness is the introduction of sustained release morphine tablets (MST-Continus in UK; MS Contin and Roxanol Sustained Release Morphine in USA). These pills have a matrix which swells as it absorbs fluid from the gastro-intestinal tract, allowing morphine to escape at a controlled rate. Consequently instead of having to take morphine every 4 h as its half-life would ordinarily dictate, dosing every 12 h (or at most every 8 h) becomes a reality. The benefits to the patient in terms of sustained comfort and the ability once more to get an undisturbed night's sleep are of real significance (Hanks and Trueman, 1983; Walsh, 1983; Foley and Inturrisi, 1987). The correct way of using this form of morphine is first to gain control of the pain with morphine elixir or immediate-release tablets given every 4 h, and once this is achieved to administer the same total daily dose of morphine in two, or at the most three, equal parts, at 12 or 8 h intervals. In the UK, sustained release morphine is available in 10, 30, 60 and 100 mg sizes. Tablets ranging in size up to 200 mg will eventually be available in the USA but, inexplicably, at present only the 30 mg tablet has been approved for sale there, so that patients requiring large doses of morphine need to take a daunting number of pills.

Although the sustained release morphine tablets are an extremely valuable innovation, the prescribing physician must use them with care in patients with abnormal gastro-intestinal physiology or anatomy Erratic absorption may occur in the case of paralytic ileus, leading alternately to loss of pain control and to significant morphine intoxication (Vere, 1984). Conversely, since the tablets are designed to release their morphine over a 12 h period, in patients whose colon has been removed, there is the real possibility that each tablet will only have time to release part of its load before entering the ileostomy bag. In this situation, patients stabilized on morphine elixir may exhibit serious loss of pain control if switched to a sustained release preparation.

Parenteral morphine and other opiates

There will inevitably be some patients for whom oral medication is not feasible, for example those with oesophageal carcinoma, or with persistent vomiting. For them, some type of parenteral administration is needed, and in most cases this will be in the form of a chronic intravenous or subcutaneous infusion. Intravenous infusions have obvious difficulties in that if peripheral veins are used, access may be lost because of displacement of the needle or venous thrombosis. These problems are sometimes avoided by administering the drug into a central vein via a Hickman catheter, but quite apart from the special skills needed for its insertion, it requires meticulous attention to prevent sepsis.

An alternative approach is chronic subcutaneous infusion, using a butterfly needle (which anyone can place) attached to a small portable pump. Although the subcutaneous route has some advantages, it also has problems of its own. For example, the volume of fluid which can be infused into the subcutaneous tissues it not infinitely large, and given the limited solubility of morphine this can restrict its usefulness. Local irritation commonly occurs at the site of the infusion, necessitating replacement of the needle every few days. Sometimes a local reaction walls off the infusion site so that the solution is confined to a loculated area, with correspondingly poor absorption of the opiate.

There are now a variety of infusion pumps on the market. One, devoid of moving parts, employs an elastomeric balloon which will deliver a solution at a predetermined and unalterable rate as the distended reservoir contracts. A widely used but fairly simple mechanical device to which a standard disposable syringe is attached is the Graesby syringe driver (Oliver, 1985), sold as the Infusaid External Pump in the USA. This device allows the drug to be infused at a variable rate, and has provision for the administration of an extra bolus dose if needed to control breakthrough pain. At a higher price, pumps of great sophistication can be obtained, such as the Pharmacia-Deltec CADD/PCA device. This goes to great lengths to control the patient's access to the drug. The solution is contained in a locked compartment in the body of the pump. The pump is programmed to deliver a wide range of infusion rates, and also has provision for the administration of a preset number of bolus doses by the patient. The number of bolus doses per hour and the time interval between them are also programmed into the pump by the physician, and the pump's controlling circuitry is then electronically 'locked' to prevent unauthorized alteration by the patient.

No matter which pump is used, as a practical matter, it is rarely possible to infuse more than 2.0 ml/h into a subcutaneous site. For most patients, given that the maximum concentration of morphine readily available is 35 mg/ml, this is adequate. However there are some who need more. The greater solubility of diamorphine (in the UK), or of hydromorphone (in the USA) may lead to these drugs being more widely used in this situation in the future.

Infusion of opiates directly into the central nervous system

Direct administration of opiates into the CNS, both acutely and by means of chronic infusion devices, has also attracted attention over the last 7–8 years. Opiates have been infused into both the epidural and intrathecal spaces (Cousins and Mather, 1984), as well as into the cerebral ventricles (Lobato et al, 1985). Opiates have important advantages over local anaesthetics in the context of spinal injection, being selective in their action. In contrast, agents such as lignocaine (lidocaine) obliterate motor, sensory and autonomic functions indiscriminately. Moreover in the event of an accidental overdose, there is no pharmacological antagonist to the local anaesthetics. This is not to say that opiates are devoid of problems. The most serious, a consequence of rostral spread in the cerebrospinal fluid, is respiratory depression. It is important to remember that this depression may be most marked some 7–10 h after the spinal injection, so that prolonged observation is necessary. Sedation, nausea, pruritis and urinary retention also commonly occur. With more prolonged administration, unwanted tolerance may develop, but this can be overcome by briefly substituting a local anaesthetic agent for 24–48 h, to allow the opiate receptors to recover. Surgical techniques have been developed to keep epidural and intrathecal catheters in place for prolonged periods of time (Poletti et al, 1981), though dislodging of catheters remains a potential problem, as does sepsis. In an attempt to reduce the latter, completely implantable devices have been developed.

The indications for direct administration of opiates into the central nervous system are relatively few, since most patients can be managed so well with oral, sub-cutaneous or intravenous agents. However the very high concentration of opiates which can be achieved is occasionally useful, although the therapeutic window remains very narrow.

Neurosurgical techniques for the relief of pain

With increasing pharmacological sophistication the need for neurosurgical techniques is declining. Moreover, particularly in patients who survive for several months, any neuroablative procedure carries with it the possibility of recurrent pain because of deafferentation. In the short term however, regional nerve blocks (*e.g.* of an intercostal nerve, using either chemicals such as phenol, or a cryoprobe to freeze the nerve), and chemical sympathectomies (*e.g.* a coeliac plexus block) are all well-established techniques for providing short- to medium-term relief from fairly localized sources of pain. Radio frequency lesions of the spinothalamic tract (cordotomy) can be produced using a percutaneous approach, and these may be very effective in providing relief from strictly unilateral pain below the level of C5. The method is well described by Lipton (1984). For patients with painful lesions above the level of C5, an alternative exists in the form of stereotaxic neuroablation of various tracts. The results of this approach are moderately good for patients with nociceptive pain (Tasker, 1984b), but interestingly, the results in patients with deafferentation pain have not been as encouraging. Conceivably this is because deafferentation involves a degree of 'denervation hypersensitivity' in central structures which will not be lessened by neuroablation distal to them. This putative mechanism may also explain why patients with deafferentation gain relief at least temporarily from parenteral barbiturates and local anaesthetics (Tasker, 1984a).

Other techniques which are more controversial and somewhat unproven include pituitary ablation by alcohol injection (Lipton, 1979), and the stereotaxic stimulation of the parabrachial area of the brain (Katayama et al, 1985) that apparently activates cholinergic rather than opiate-dependent mechanisms. This latter approach is exciting not so much because of the possibility of expanding the application of neurosurgical techniques to pain control, but because it suggests the possibility of other mechanisms which might be susceptible to pharmacological manipulation.

POTENTIAL FUTURE DEVELOPMENTS

The recognition of the heterogeneity of opiate receptors has spurred the development of a variety of agents specific for each of them, in the hopes of producing a drug which, while retaining analgesic properties, will be lacking in the limiting side-effects such as sedation, tolerance, constipation or nausea which characterize the opiates currently in use. Intense studies of enkephalin and endorphin analogues are also under way for the same reasons.

So far, no clinically accepted compound has been developed, but there are several interesting developments. Meptazinol has been reported to be selective for μ_1-receptors (which mediate analgesia) (Spiegel and Pasternak, 1984). Relative lack of dependency and respiratory depression *may* be due to a lower μ_2-potency, but the issue is complicated by the fact that meptazinol also has anticholinesterase properties (Galli, 1985; Wali, 1986). The whole area of cholinergic agents as analgesics is ripe for exploration.

DADLE (D-alanine-D-leucine-enkephalin), a δ-opiate receptor agonist, has been reported to produce analgesia in situations where tolerance to morphine (a μ-agonist) has developed (Moulin et al, 1985).

Compounds active on the κ-receptor have also attracted attention since it has been claimed that stimulation of such receptors produces as much pain relief as stimulation of μ-receptors by morphine, but with less dependence, sedation and respiratory depression. Pentazocine, butorphanol and the experimental compounds U50488 and xorphanol are being evaluated in this respect.

As a final possibility, which to date has received no attention, with the advent of opiates of extremely high potency, the possibility of developing a transdermal patch like those used for hyoscine (scopolamine) and clonidine should be considered. Opiates such as fentanyl and etorphine would seem to be obvious candidates for such an approach.

SUMMARY

In recent years, the complexity of the mechanisms involved in pain perception have slowly been appreciated. It is now known that nociceptive impulses arriving from the periphery are subject to control by segmental interneurons, and by descending fibres from higher centres, which may block their rostral transmission. The mechanisms involved in this modulation are being intensively investigated in a quest for drugs which can mimic the endogenous analgesic mechanisms. Analogues of enkephalins and endorphins show promise in certain respects. Identification of sub-types of opiate receptors has also raised the possibility of producing drugs which retain the analgesic action of morphine while losing the undesirable side-effects. Recent developments have also included new ways of delivering old drugs. Foremost among these has been the advent of sustained release morphine tablets, for these have provided a major advance in the quality of life of many of the terminally ill. Other methods such as ventricular or epidural or intrathecal infusion of opiates, and a variety of neurosurgical techniques, have also been considered.

Despite all the recent advances in knowledge, the management of pain in the terminally ill throughout the world remains a disgrace. What is needed now is not a stunning new understanding of pain pharmacology, but the consistent and rational application of what we already know. History will judge us harshly if we continue to fail to meet even this modest goal.

REFERENCES

Baines M & Kirkham SR (1984) Carcinoma involving bone and soft tissue. In Wall PD & Melzack R (eds) *Textbook of Pain*, pp 453–459. London: Churchill Livingstone.

Basbaum AI (1985) Functional analysis of the cytochemistry of the spinal dorsal horn. *Advances in Pain Research and Therapy* **9:** 149–175.

Bonica JJ (1985) Treatment of cancer pain: current status and future needs. *Advances in Pain Research and Therapy* **9:** 589–616.

Chahl LA (1979) Pain induced by inflammatory mediators. In Beers RF & Bennett EG (eds) *Mechanisms of Pain and Analgesic Compounds*, pp 273–284. New York: Raven Press.

Cousins MJ & Mather LE (1984) Intrathecal and epidural administration of opioids. *Anesthesiology* **61:** 276–310.

Foley KM (1985) Pharmacologic approaches to cancer pain management. *Advances in Pain Research and Therapy* **9:** 629–653.

Foley KM (1987) Pain syndromes in patients with cancer. *Medical Clinics of North America* **71:** 169–184.

Foley KM & Inturrisi CE (1987) Analgesic drug therapy in cancer pain: principles and practice. *Medical Clinics of North America* **71:** 207–232.

Galli A (1985) Inhibition of cholinesterases by the opioid analgesic meptazinol. *Biochemical Pharmacology* **34:** 1579–1581.

Hanks GW & Trueman T (1983) Controlled-release morphine tablets are effective in twice-daily dosage in chronic cancer pain. *Royal Society of Medicine. International Congress and Symposium Series* **64:** 103–105.

Katayama Y, Tsubokawa T, Hirayama T et al (1985) Pain relief following stimulation of the pontomesencephalic parabrachial region in humans: brain site for non-opiate-mediated pain control. *Applied Neurophysiology* **48:** 1579–1581.

Liebeskind JC & Melzack R (1987) The international pain foundation: Meeting a need for education in pain management. *Pain* **30:** 1–2.

Lipton S (1979) *The Control of Chronic Pain*, pp 104–107. London: Edward Arnold.

Lipton S (1984) Percutaneous cordotomy In Wall PD & Melzack R (eds) *Textbook of Pain*, pp 632–638. London: Churchill Livingstone.

Lobato RD, Madrid JL, Fatela LV et al (1985) Analgesia elicited by low-dose intraventricular morphine in terminal cancer patients. *Advances in Pain Research and Therapy* **9:** 673–681.

Moulin DE, Max MB, Kaiko RF et al (1985) The analgesic efficacy of intrathecal D-ala^2-D-leu^5-enkephalin in cancer patients with chronic pain. *Pain* **23:** 213–221.

Oliver DJ (1985) The use of the syringe driver in terminal care. *British Journal of Clinical Pharmacology* **20:** 515–516.

Payne R (1987) Anatomy, physiology and neuropharmacology of cancer pain. *Medical Clinics of North America* **71:** 153–167.

Poletti CE, Cohen AM, Todd DP et al (1981) Cancer pain relieved by long term epidural morphine with permanent indwelling system for self administration. *Journal of Neurosurgery* **55:** 581–584.

Pomeranz B, Wall P & Weber WV (1968) Cord cells responding to fine myelinated afferents and skin. *Journal of Physiology* **199:** 511–532.

Saunders C (1984) The philosophy of terminal care. In Saunders C (ed.) *The Management of Terminal Malignant Disease*, pp 232–241. London: Edward Arnold.

Spiegel K & Pasternak GW (1984) Meptazinol: a novel μ_1 selective opioid analgesic. *Journal of Pharmacology and Experimental Therapeutics* **228:** 414–419.

Taira N & Nakano T (1974) Is intra-arterial 5-hydroxytryptamine a potent algogenic substance in the dog? *European Journal of Pharmacology* **25:** 113–116.

Tasker RR (1984a) Deafferentation. In Wall PD & Melzack R (eds) *Textbook of Pain*, pp 119–132. London: Churchill Livingstone.

Tasker RR (1984b) Stereotaxic surgery. In Wall PD & Melzack R (eds) *Textbook of Pain*, pp 639–655. London: Churchill-Livingstone.

Twycross RG (1984) Relief of pain. In Saunders C (ed.) *The Management of Terminal Disease*, pp 64–90. London: Edward Arnold.

Twycross RG & Lack SA (1984) *Therapeutics in Terminal Cancer*, p 9. London: Pitman.

Vere D (1984) Death from sustained release morphine sulphate. *Lancet* **i:** 1477.

Wali FA (1986) On the cholinergic component of action of meptazinol. *Acta Physiologica et Pharmacologica Latinoamericana* **36:** 77–87.
Wall PD (1985) Cancer pain: neurogenic mechanisms. *Advances in Pain Research and Therapy* **9:** 575–587.
Wall PD & Sweet WH (1967) Temporary abolition of pain in man. *Science* **155:** 108–109.
Walsh TD, Baster R, Bowman K & Leber R (1981) High dose morphine and respiratory function in chronic cancer pain. *Pain* (supplement **1**): 39.
Walsh TD (1983) A controlled study of MST Continus tablets for chronic pain in advanced cancer. *Society of Medicine. International Congress and Symposium Series* **64:** 99–102.
Woolf CJ (1983) Evidence for a central component of post-injury pain hypersensitivity. *Nature* **306:** 686–688.
Woolf CJ (1985) Functional plasticity of the flexor withdrawal reflex in the rat following peripheral tissue injury. *Advances in Pain Research and Therapy* **9:** 193–201.

11

The management of malignant spinal cord compression

SUSAN CLOSS
THELMA D. BATES

Acute spinal cord compression due to malignant disease is a medical emergency, and the key to successful management is early diagnosis and prompt treatment. All too often the diagnosis is made too late for useful treatment. It is essential that oncologists, general practitioners and hospice physicians are alert to the possibility of the syndrome in patients complaining of back pain, especially those with bone metastases, whether or not there is radiological evidence of vertebral collapse. As neurological recovery is inversely related to the degree of initial impairment, it is vital that the diagnosis is made when there is minimal loss of function. Once a patient becomes unable to walk, the chance of restoring mobility by whatever means is small.

ANATOMY OF SPINAL CORD COMPRESSION

The spinal cord includes the origins of many efferent pathways and the terminations of many of the afferent pathways. These are carried in 31 pairs of spinal nerves, each with a dorsal and a ventral root. The cord extends from the upper border of the atlas to the lower border of the first lumbar vertebra but the lower level is subject to some anatomical variation which is of clinical significance. It may end as high as the lower border of the 12th thoracic vertebra or as low as the upper border of the third lumbar vertebra. The cord terminates in a leash of nerve roots, the cauda equina, which traverse the subarachnoid space to leave the spinal canal through their intervertebral formina. The surface markings of the nerve segments are shown in Table 1.

The motor path

After decussation in the medulla, the corticospinal (pyramidal) tracts pass caudally in the lateral columns of the spinal cord, terminating in the anterior horn cells on the same side. Approximately one third of the motor fibres

Table 1. The surface markings of the nerve segments.

Vertebral spine position	Corresponding cord segment
C6	7th cervical
T4	6th thoracic
T10	1st lumbar
T11	3rd lumbar
T12	1st sacral

from the cerebrum do not cross in the medulla but pass down the same side of the spinal cord in the anterior column. These too terminate in the anterior horn cells. Interlinking of the neurones within the anterior grey column accounts for the observation that fibres of the corticospinal tracts correspond with groups of muscles and not with individual muscles.

The lateral column and anterior horn cells are the elements most sensitive to compression, as there is a 'watershed' between venous drainage areas here. If the corticospinal tract alone is damaged, extensor hypertonicity is the result, but if the reticulospinal tracts are also involved then flexor spasm predominates. Thus, slowly progressive cord compression first produces a paresis and eventually paraplegia. Damage to the anterior horn cells in the ventral grey matter produces lower motor neurone signs of wasting, weakness, flaccidity and areflexia. The latter is usually a late manifestation of progressive lower motor neurone damage. Fascicular twitching may also be present.

Compression of the cauda equina results in lower motor neurone lesions in the lumbar and sacral nerves supplying the lower limbs, bladder and rectum. Interruption of the reflex arc of the bladder (S2, S3 and S4) results in retention of urine.

The sensory path

All sensory fibres from the limbs and trunk enter the spinal cord by the dorsal roots. The sensations of light touch and proprioception from the ipsilateral side are carried in the dorsal columns. Compression of these afferent fibres causes a sensation of a tight band around the trunk (girdle pain), pins and needles and numbness. Occasionally, cervical tumours may cause tingling or electric shock sensations in the trunk or limbs by pressure on this area.

The lateral spinothalamic tract carries sensations of pain and temperature from the opposite side of the body. The decussation of these afferent fibres occurs two or three segments higher than the nerve root entry. Compression of this tract can cause a variety of symptoms such as burning, tingling, sensations of hot and cold water on the skin, or jabs of pain.

AETIOLOGY OF MALIGNANT CORD COMPRESSION

Compression of spinal nerve tissue can be extrinsic or intrinsic. Extrinsic lesions which produce pressure effects on the cord may be extradural tumours such as metastatic carcinomas or lymphomas, or less commonly subdural lesions such as meningiomas. Intrinsic tumours, astrocytomas or ependymomas, are much rarer causes. Meningeal deposits of carcinoma (especially from breast), lymphoma and leukaemia may, on rare occasions, spread in the cerebrospinal fluid and cause intradural deposits.

Tumours can themselves cause direct compression of the spinal cord (*non-structural or tumoral compression*) or cause indirect compression by local destruction of the vertebrae which then compress the cord (*structural compression*). Structural damage to vertebrae producing deformity and collapse occurs in malignant diseases which have a propensity for bone metastases, i.e. carcinomas of the bronchus, breast, kidney, thyroid and prostate. Multiple myeloma also frequently involves the vertebrae and causes bone destruction. Tumours may also erode bone and gain entry into the extradural space by direct extension from the vertebra. Any part of the vertebra may be involved but even with total destruction and collapse of the bone matrix, the intervertebral discs are spared. This radiological feature helps to differentiate between malignant disease and infective conditions: the latter usually involve the disc as well.

Malignant lymphomas, in contrast, compress the spinal cord by direct spread through intervertebral foramina from mediastinal or retroperitoneal lymph nodes (non-structural compression). Tumour in the extradural space can occur in any position and the location is important for the surgeon; posteriorly placed deposits are considered by some to be more accessible than those situated anteriorly (Brice and McKissoch, 1965; Hall and Mackay, 1973).

The anatomical distribution of epidural metastases is similar in most series—approximately 70% in the thoracic spine, 30% in the lumbar and 10% in the cervical spine (Torma, 1957; White et al, 1971). It is uncertain whether this distribution reflects a predeliction for metastases to involve the thoracic spine or whether it reflects the proportion of the spinal column occupied by the thoracic vertebrae. Multiple levels of cord compression are not uncommon, and in a series by Gilbert et al (1978) 22 of 130 cases (19%) had cord compression at more than one site.

Most studies show that carcinomas of the bronchus, breast, prostate or kidney are the commonest primary tumours producing spinal cord compression (Table 2). Lymphomas appear to have a high incidence according to the literature but it is possible that, with more effective radical treatment of this disease, the incidence of spinal cord compression as a complication may now be less than it was. In Black's review of the literature (1979), 9% of cases of spinal cord compression were due to metastases from an unidentified primary.

Some malignancies have a predeliction to metastasize to the vertebral column or extradural space. Barron et al (1959) showed in an autopsy series on patients who had died from malignant disease, that multiple myeloma was the tumour most likely to involve the vertebrae (14% of 21 patients), followed by prostatic carcinoma (10% of 40 patients) and renal carcinoma (8% of 40 patients). Surprisingly, vertebral involvement by carcinoma of the bronchus and breast in this study was only 5% and 7% respectively.

Table 2. Spinal metastases: location of the primary tumour in 1038 clinical cases, pooled from literature 1957–1978.

Location of primary tumour	Cases of spinal metastases (%)	
Lung	15	Approximately half of all cases
Breast	14	
Lymphoma	11	
Unknown	9	
Sarcoma	8	
Myeloma	7	
Prostate	7	
Kidney	6	
Gastro-intestinal	4	
Miscellaneous	18	

From Black (1979), with permission.

However, Cobb et al (1977) showed, in a very large retrospective series of 12 000 patients with carcinoma of the breast, that 20% proved to have vertebral metastases at autopsy, although only 2% had had neurological problems due to cord compression.

Although the presence of spinal cord compression usually denotes advanced disease, in 8% of patients spinal cord compression was a presenting feature (Gilbert et al, 1978). In a recent study at St Christopher's Hospice, spinal cord compression was the first evidence of malignant disease in seven of 46 patients (Closs, unpublished data). On the other hand, there may be a prolonged latent period between the diagnosis of cancer and the development of spinal cord compression, and Cobb et al (1977) record one patient with carcinoma of the breast who developed spinal cord compression 19 years after the original diagnosis.

In most studies there is a slightly higher incidence of spinal cord compression in males. The average age corresponds to that period in life when there is a greater incidence of cancer, i.e. 40–65 years, the peak being 50–60 years.

DIAGNOSIS OF SPINAL CORD COMPRESSION

Early diagnosis of cord compression is essential in order to facilitate early treatment—neurological recovery being related to the degree of pre-treatment neurological impairment. Therefore, a delay of days, and possibly hours, may be critical. An accurate history of the timing of events, the sequence of progression, the current status of the patient and the histology of the primary tumour are all of importance and will influence the mode of treatment and the likely outcome.

Symptoms and signs

During the development of spinal cord compression the common sequence of events is back pain, motor dysfunction, paraesthesia and sensory loss, followed by sphincter dysfunction. It is worth noting that motor and sensory symptoms may be less obvious in patients confined to bed. Onset may be acute or insidious, and pain may precede other symptoms by days or even years. Involvement of the cauda equina characteristically causes 'saddle' anaesthesia, loss of sphincter sensation and urinary incontinence. Lesions above the level of C5, fortunately rare, may give rise to respiratory failure.

In the series of Gilbert et al (1978) pain was the initial symptom in 96% of patients and this preceded other symptoms by five days to two years. At diagnosis, 76% had some weakness or disturbance of gait, 15% were paraplegic, 51% complained of numbness or paraesthesia and 57% had sphincter disturbances.

Pain and spinal tenderness

Pain is the commonest presenting symptom and backache must never be disregarded in patients with malignant disease. Pain may be local or radicular. Local pain is more common and usually corresponds fairly well to the site of the lesion. It is not infrequently associated with unilateral or bilateral radicular pain. Thoracic deposits produce a 'girdle pain' which is always of bilateral distribution, whereas cervical or lumbar deposits produce unilateral or bilateral pain in the limbs. Pain due to vertebral disease is usually a constant intolerable deep-seated aching pain, while nerve root pain is severe and sharp, described as being like an electric shock or a searing knife. These pains are not relieved by mild analgesics and are usually exacerbated by movement, coughing or sneezing. With slowly growing tumours compressing the sensory pathways, pain may be described as burning or cramp-like. Vertebral tenderness is not always present but when elicited is a useful physical sign of location.

Motor dysfunction

Early motor symptoms often complained of, but sometimes disregarded, are of tripping up, leg stiffness, difficulty in going upstairs or getting on the bus, and slowness of gait. The danger is that all of these symptoms are easily explained away as acceptable and inevitable symptoms in a patient with malignant disease. Signs of spasticity may be missed by over-vigorous examination of the tone of the legs when employing passive flexion and extension of the knees. Weakness is also difficult to define because it occurs in the flexor groups in the lower limbs at first and is sometimes not noted until paraplegia has supervened and there is no voluntary movement left to test.

With paraplegia due to rapid cord compression there is a flaccid paralysis, often with a distended bladder and absent reflexes, but with more gradual development of compression hyper-reflexia may be present. A spinal cord lesion situated at or above the C5 segment produces quadriplegia. If the arms are totally spared, the lesion lies below T1, while for lesions at T1 the small muscles of the hand are affected (plus evidence of Horner's syndrome).

Sensory loss

Sensory complaints are rare as presenting symptoms but common sensory symptoms at diagnosis are paraesthesia, numbness, coldness and loss of balance. The sensory levels are generally within one or two vertebral bodies of the site of the lesion. Sensory loss to pin-prick, vibration and position tend to parallel that of motor weakness, although some sensation to firm touch may remain in grossly paraplegic patients. Lesions of the conus medullaris and the cauda equina are associated with a 'saddle' anaesthesia—a loss of cutaneous sensibility in the perineum, buttocks, back of thigh, leg and sole of the foot.

Bladder and bowel dysfunction

Sphincter function is often preserved until cord compression is well advanced. Early sphincter disturbances include hesitancy and precipitancy of micturition and these generally precede urinary retention with overflow incontinence and severe constipation with spurious diarrhoea. In compression of the conus medullaris and cauda equina, sphincter dysfunction is associated with 'saddle' anaesthesia.

INVESTIGATIONS

An urgent plain X-ray of the whole spine is mandatory. It may reveal bone destruction, loss of a pedicle or vertebral body collapse (usually sparing the intervertebral disc) at one or more levels. It may also reveal a soft tissue mass adjacent to the vertebrae.

An urgent myelogram gives valuable information concerning the site and extent of the compression. Lumbar puncture is contra-indicated, except as part of a myelogram, as it may exacerbate compression.

A computerized tomography (CT) scan or magnetic resonance imaging (MRI) can be helpful in demonstrating an associated soft tissue mass. But this must not delay treatment, and is only helpful if immediately available.

DIFFERENTIAL DIAGNOSIS OF SPINAL CORD COMPRESSION

In a patient with malignant disease who complains of back pain with or without any of the other signs and symptoms of spinal cord compression, there should always be a high level of suspicion, and all neurological symptoms should be taken as features of cord compression until proved otherwise. Particularly easy to overlook are the few patients whose presenting symptoms of their malignancy are those of incipient spinal cord compression.

Reasonable certainty of the diagnosis is established by the presence of radiological signs of vertebral erosion or collapse. Previous trauma, crush fractures due to osteoporosis, tuberculosis, pyogenic infection and syphilis can also cause vertebral erosion and collapse but, as noted above, the intervertebral disc remains intact in malignant disease but is often eroded in the case of infective disease. Prolapsed intervertebral discs, severe scoliosis or kyphosis may also produce spinal cord or cauda equina disturbances, as can osteoarthritis, spondylolisthesis, herpes zoster and primary neurological diseases such as multiple sclerosis and motor neurone disease.

Prompt myelography is indicated for any patient in whom there is a suspicion of spinal cord or nerve root compression. In patients with malignant disease and a normal myelogram, there is a possibility of meningeal carcinomatosis (when malignant cells in the CSF will confirm the diagnosis), a malignant neuropathy or myopathy or radiation damage of the spinal cord.

MANAGEMENT OF SPINAL CORD COMPRESSION

Prevention

Acute spinal cord compression can often be anticipated in patients with bone metastases and a moderate degree of vertebral collapse, even in the absence of pain or other symptoms. In such cases, a course of prophylactic radiotherapy can do no harm and may prevent this distressing syndrome. Such treatment should always be accompanied by practical advice on bending, twisting and lifting and the provision of a spinal support corset if appropriate. Even in the presence of a normal radiograph, a patient with a persistent backache which is getting worse (particularly a patient suffering from a malignant lymphoma or melanoma) should be considered at an early stage for referral for a myelogram to exclude epidural deposits. It is not advisable to delay treatment until the development of neurological signs.

In the presence of a potentially unstable spine, decisions have to be made concerning restriction of mobility and the need for operative spinal stabilization. These decisions will be influenced by the patient's general condition and the prognosis. Few would deprive a terminally ill patient of mobility, and occasionally risks have to be taken. The help and advice of a physiotherapist are invaluable at this time.

Treatment

It is vital to stress that acute spinal cord compression is a medical emergency and that the key to success is early diagnosis and prompt treatment. Treatment involves urgent decompression of the cord by either surgery or radiotherapy or a combination of both. On rare occasions, chemotherapy is an option.

Initially, all patients should receive corticosteroids to reduce spinal cord oedema. Especially in the early case, this will result in a reduction of pain, and in some, temporary neurological recovery. The optimal dosage has not been established. Dexamethasone 16 mg daily in divided doses has been recommended (Gilbert et al, 1978) and is a frequent prescription. Marshall and Langfit (1977) use doses up to 40 mg daily for patients who show no benefit from lower doses, while Greenberg et al (1980) advise 100 mg daily for three days followed by rapidly progressive reduction.

Surgical decompression

Surgical decompression has the advantages of providing rapid decompression and also the opportunity to explore the extent of the tumour and obtain histology (important when the primary site is unknown). Only surgery can relieve structural compression and that caused by radioresistant tumours. The disadvantages are the high operative morbidity, an operative mortality of 3–13%, and a worsening of neurological status in about 12% of cases (Black, 1979). Poor results are obtained in patients who have already progressed to paraplegia and bladder dysfunction (Törmä, 1957; Barron et al, 1959; White et al, 1971) but Larson et al (1961) pointed out that although surgical decompression may not restore neurological function in many patients, it may arrest progression and preserve remaining function.

While opinions vary, most would agree that the indications for surgical decompression are rapidly progressing compression in a relatively fit patient, a complete block, a structural compression and a tumour which is non-sensitive to radiotherapy. It is also the treatment of choice for high cervical cord lesions and for cases where the precise cause of spinal cord compression is unknown.

Surgery usually involves a wide laminectomy and removal of sufficient epidural tumour to relieve cord compression (White et al, 1971). Recently an anterior decompression with spinal stabilization has been described with seemingly very much better results (Siegal et al, 1982). Whatever the surgical approach for the unstable spine, spinal fixation by autogenous bone graft, Harrington's rods or acrylic fusion will be necessary (Gunn et al, 1974; Harrington, 1981).

Post-operative radiotherapy

Total eradication of epidural metastases by surgery is virtually impossible and therefore post-operative radiotherapy is recommended for most patients. It improves the functional result, gives better pain control and reduces the probability of local recurrence when compared with laminectomy alone (Findlay, 1984). The volume to be irradiated is decided with the neurosurgeon and treatment is started as soon as the wound has healed.

Decompression by radiotherapy

There are no valid randomized prospective studies comparing the effectiveness of surgical versus radiation decompression, but clearly, radiotherapy does not have the immediacy of effect of surgery, nor could it restore stability to collapsed vertebrae. Patients most suitable for management with radiotherapy are those with a gradual onset and progression of symptoms, non-structural compression due to a tumour which is radiosensitive (lymphomas, myeloma, leukaemic deposits) and lesions of the cauda equina.

Radiotherapy should be started immediately, together with concurrent corticosteroid therapy (dexamethasone tablets 4 mg every 6 h). A direct posterior field is used which extends two vertebral levels above and below the lesion, and a dose approaching the level of spinal cord tolerance is given.

Conventional radiotherapy is given in a dose of 2 Gy daily delivered five times weekly to a total dose of 25–40 Gy (Khan et al, 1967; Friedman et al, 1976). In an experimental spinal epidural tumour model in rats, Rubin (1969) showed that higher daily doses were more effective than low doses. On the basis of these findings, others have given 5 Gy daily for 3 days followed by 4 days rest and then five daily doses of 3 Gy (30 Gy in eight treatments over 12 days) (Greenberg et al, 1980; Tomita et al, 1983). The author's technique (TB) is to give 30 Gy in six treatments over 18 days).

Choice of the method of decompression

The choice of the method of decompression will depend on several factors:

General condition of the patient. Not all patients are fit for surgical decompression, and the presence of hypercalcaemia or a compromised bone marrow following chemotherapy may make surgery more hazardous.

Duration, severity and tempo of the clinical picture. A rapid onset and progression of symptoms and the presence of a myelographic complete block suggest the need for urgent surgical decompression. However, most patients who are already paraplegic are likely to remain so after decompression, whether it is carried out by surgery or radiotherapy.

Level of cord compression. A high cervical cord lesion with the possibility of respiratory failure necessitates urgent surgical decompression rather than risk the delayed benefits of radiotherapy. On the other hand, a cauda equina lesion can reasonably be treated by radiotherapy.

Multiple levels of compression are generally best treated by radiotherapy because of the magnitude of the surgery necessary.

Cause of the compression. Structural compression due to severe vertebral collapse or compression fracture cannot be relieved by radiotherapy. Only surgical decompression and spinal stabilization can achieve this. On the other hand, for non-structural compression due to epidural tumour deposits, radiotherapy is an option.

Radiosensitivity of the tumour. Highly radiosensitive tumours include lymphomas, leukaemic deposits, myelomas, neuroblastomas and Ewing's tumour. When these tumours produce gradual non-structural cord compression, radiotherapy alone is considered to be the treatment of choice (Friedman et al, 1976). On the other hand, radiotherapy is not appropriate for radioresistant tumours (melanomas, renal carcinomas and sarcomas) or for patients where the tissues have been previously irradiated. Carcinomas of the breast, bronchus and prostate are moderately radiosensitive and their management will be influenced more by the other factors listed above.

Chemosensitivity of the tumour. In general, cytotoxic chemotherapy plays a secondary role in patients with spinal cord compression, but it may have a primary role in a few chemosensitive tumours such as a testicular teratoma, Hodgkin's disease and non-Hodgkin's lymphoma (Bruckman and Bloomer, 1978).

RESULTS OF DECOMPRESSION

The aim of treatment is to restore neurological function—to allow the patient to walk, to have control over his bladder and bowel and to relieve pain. The success of treatment is largely dependent on the pre-treatment status; adverse features being rapid neurological deterioration, established paraplegia, bladder dysfunction and compression at several levels.

It is difficult to make comparisons between surgical and radiation series because selection of cases has taken place. In a critical review of the literature since 1960, Findlay (1984) found that only 25% of the 1816 cases presented while still able to walk. Overall in the series, the results of treatment by any method (surgery, surgery plus radiotherapy or radiotherapy alone) were disappointing and showed that only 35% of patients retained or returned to the ability to walk, while some 20–25% sustained major neurological deterioration. The best results were obtained in the sub-group presenting while still able to walk, with 48%, 67% and 79% remaining ambulatory following surgery, surgery plus radiotherapy and radiotherapy alone respectively.

In a series of 79 patients with epidural metastases producing a complete spinal block who were treated by radiotherapy alone at the Sloan Kettering Institute (Tomita et al, 1983), only two patients improved and 11 non-paraplegics became paraplegic. Nevertheless, 70% of the patients who were able to walk with or without assistance pre-operatively, retained that ability.

Little mention is made in the literature of preservation of sphincter control. Loss of sphincter control is generally a late event and in those patients who remain non-ambulatory, treatment could be said to have benefited them provided they do not deteriorate further and lose their sphincter control. Certainly from a patient's point of view, such a loss is never acceptable.

The literature tends to emphasize the length of survival, which is usually shorter in carcinoma of the lung than in carcinoma of the breast. This emphasis would seem to be of limited importance in the palliation and prevention of such distressing symptoms. It merely serves to discourage early and appropriate aggressive treatment of patients with a limited life expectancy.

A more positive attitude to the treatment of this difficult and distressing condition is important. Although the results of treatment in terms of neurological recovery are often disappointing, merely to halt progress of the condition, especially in an ambulatory state with sphincters intact, is worthwhile even if it is only for a relatively short time.

REFERENCES

Barron KD, Hirano A, Araki S & Terry RD (1959) Experiences with metastatic neoplasms involving the spinal cord. *Neurology* (Minneapolis) **9:** 91–106.

Black P (1979) Spinal metastasis: current status and recommended guidelines for management. *Neurosurgery* **5:** 726–746.

Brice J & McKissock W (1965) Surgical treatment of malignant epidural spinal tumours. *British Medical Journal* **1:** 1341–1344.

Bruckman JE & Bloomer WD (1978) Management of spinal cord compression. *Seminars in Oncology* **5:** 135–140.

Cobb CA, Leavens ME & Eckles N (1977) Indications for non-operative treatment of spinal cord compression due to breast cancer. *Journal of Neurosurgery* **47:** 653–658.

Findlay GFG (1984) Adverse effects of the management of malignant spinal cord compression. *Journal of Neurology, Neurosurgery and Psychiatry* **47:** 761–768.

Friedman M, Kim TH & Panahon AM (1976) Spinal cord compression in malignant lymphoma: treatment and results. *Cancer* **37:** 1485–1491.

Gilbert RW, Kim Jae-Ho & Posner JB (1978) Epidural spinal cord compression from metastatic tumour: diagnosis and treatment. *Annals of Neurology* **3:** 40–51.

Greenberg HS, Kim Jae-Ho & Posner JB (1980) Epidural spinal cord compression from metastatic tumour: results with a new treatment protocol. *Annals of Neurology* **8:** 361–366.

Gunn D, Tupper J & Muller M (1974) Decompression and immediate stabilisation of the spine in patients suffering from malignant disease. *Journal of Bone and Joint Surgery*, American Volume **56:** 1767.

Hall AJ & Mackay NNS (1973) The results of laminectomy for compression of the cord and cauda equina by extradural malignant tumour. *Journal of Bone and Joint Surgery*, British Volume **55:** 497–505.

Harrington K (1981) The use of methylmethacylate for vertebral body replacement and anterior stabilisation of pathological fracture–dislocation of the spine due to metastatic malignant disease. *Journal of Bone and Joint Surgery*, American Volume **63:** 36–46.

Khan FR, Glicksman AS, Chu FCH & Nickson JJ (1967) Treatment by radiotherapy of spinal cord compression due to extradural metastases. *Radiology* **89:** 495–500.

Larson S, Wetzel N, Brochner R & Ruge D (1961) The surgical treatment of metastatic epidural tumours. *Quarterly Bulletin of the Northwestern University Medical School* **35:** 42–44.

Marshall LF & Langfit TW (1977) Combined therapy for metastatic extradural tumours of the spine. *Cancer* **40:** 2067–2070.

Rubin P (1969) Extradural spinal cord compression by tumour: Part I. Experimental production and treatment trials. *Radiology* **93:** 1243–1248.

Siegal T, Siegal T, Robin G, Lubetzki-Kom I & Fuks Z (1982) Anterior decompression of the spine for metastatic epidural cord compression: A promising avenue of therapy? *Annals of Neurology* **11:** 28–34.

Tomita T, Gaicich JH & Sundaresan N (1983) Radiation therapy for spinal epidural metastases with complete block. *Acta Radiologica Oncology* **22:** 135–143.

Törmä T (1957) Malignant tumours of the spine and the spinal extradural space. A study based on 250 histologically verified cases. *Acta Chirurgica Scandinavica* **225** (supplement): 1–176.

White WA, Patterson RH & Bergland RM (1971) Role of surgery in the treatment of spinal cord compression by metastatic neoplasms. *Cancer* **27:** 558–561.

12

Knowing when not to treat

BASIL A. STOLL

Until 25 years ago medical science could offer little active treatment to the patient with distressing symptoms in cancer. Since then the position has been reversed and there is now a confusingly wide choice of new agents for treatment and sophisticated machines for investigation, therapy and life support. As a result there are many occasions when a compassionate physician needs to deliberately restrain himself from advising unnecessary investigation or unsuitably aggressive treatment. Eventually, too, there comes a time to discontinue nasogastric feeding, intravenous fluids or ventilation—an even harder decision.

There are two distinct assessments involved in the earlier decision. The first is whether the life expectation or the degree of benefit which can be expected from highly sophisticated investigation and treatment can justify the morbidity and poor quality of life which is often associated (the risk/benefit ratio). The second assessment is whether a doubtful degree of benefit can justify the investment of scarce or expensive resources which might be used more effectively, or might be in greater need, for another patient (the cost/benefit ratio).

The dilemma is minimal for the physician whose exclusive goal is the patient's peace of mind and physical comfort. His aim is to palliate troublesome symptoms using the least unpleasant forms of treatment and with the minimum of invasive investigations. However, the physician attempting to evaluate the potential of a new cancer treatment ceases to become a healer and becomes an investigator (Editorial, 1987). His obligation to identify the side-effects of treatment and to prove either response or its absence, often requires wearying and anxiety-provoking investigations for the patient, whose involvement in the trial is not primarily for personal benefit (Editorial, 1987). Informed consent to a clinical trial is easily obtained from a desperate patient, but is it meaningful under the circumstances?

Cancer patients with the symptoms described in previous chapters are distressed not only by the pain and discomfort arising from the symptoms, but also by anxiety as to how the new development may have changed their life expectancy. Every clinician is aware that routine investigations cause anxiety, and repeated monitoring increases fear even more. Each test is followed by questioning of the physician about the results and as to how far they have clarified the extent of danger to life. Knowing when not to over-investigate or over-treat the cancer patient is part of the art of medicine as opposed to its science.

ALLOCATION OF SCARCE RESOURCES

Clinical freedom of physicians in the UK means that they can sometimes concentrate scarce resources on a small group of patients in whom they are particularly interested and this is, of course, the basis of clinical research. However, it has recently become clear that some degree of rationing of resources is imperative at a time of increasingly sophisticated but increasingly expensive medical procedures, investigations, drugs and equipment (Klein, 1984). It is also obvious that misdirection of resources is just as important as shortage of funds in reducing the quality of medical treatment available for the whole population.

It is not being suggested that the physician selecting palliative treatment for the patient facing him should weigh the cost of one treatment against another or even to consider that the total palliative management is usually more expensive than curative treatment for the same disease. It is, however, not unreasonable to expect him to know what end-point he is aiming at in the care of that patient—palliation of existing symptoms, anticipation of likely symptoms or possible prolongation of life (as opposed to clutching at straws in order to reassure relatives or maintain hope in the patient).

The mark of the experienced physician is that he clearly distinguishes which one of these is his aim. A compassionate society should be prepared to spend more on cancer palliation than on cancer curative treatment but, at a certain level, the costs incurred in prolonging the terminal stage become disproportionate. It has been calculated that consumption of resources by cancer patients is most intense during the last two months of life (Silbermann, 1986). Is this rational?

There are basic differences between the approach of physicians in the UK and that in the USA. The former approach involves a more paternalistic attitude by the physician. He considers that he knows what is best for the patient and treats the patient more by his opinion of the need, than by patient demand. In the USA, on the other hand, the patient demands not only full information about his disease but also full involvement in decisions on management. USA attempts at cost-containment in recent years have tended to reduce relatively low profile services, such as home care and psychological support, but have left high technology usage almost untouched. A major reason is that high technology has a high profile, and the physician may worry about possible litigation if all the latest diagnostic and therapeutic measures are not utilized.

It is clear that the attitude of the USA physician arises from the unique social and political forces prevailing. Medicolegal pressure in the USA and the technological imperative (the idea that more sophisticated technology is necessarily more effective) lead the American doctor to practise more aggressive treatment, while British doctors are trained to be more conservative. For example, nearly all UK physicians agree that aggressive chemotherapy is not indicated as a routine palliative procedure in the majority of solid cancers of moderate or low sensitivity. The justification for such treatment could only be entry of a patient to a formal trial of a new arrangement of agents, which often involves expensive drugs, hospitalization and unpleasant investigations which are more relevant to the trial protocol than to the patient's benefit. Nevertheless, there is considerable pressure to enter patients into trials of new regimens; this includes pressures from relatives to do something active, naive optimism that advanced solid cancers resistant to other treatment may unexpectedly be arrested, and a desire to maintain the role of an up-to-date clinician. In the pursuit of such aims the patient may be offered expensive hospital treatment but denied adequate experienced care at home (Rees, 1985).

Because of different attitudes to these questions, patients with advanced cancer may be treated very differently between one institution and another, between one physician and another and between one country and another. These differences in treatment practice result from different goals which can be summarized as follows:

1. Using aggressive treatment for palliation only when symptoms appear. Individual modalities are used sequentially and are saved up as far as possible.
2. Using aggressive combination treatments either in the context of a clinical trial or in the unproven belief that life may be prolonged.
3. Treating for 'supportive reasons' in order to maintain hope in the patient or relatives.

Because of the rapidly rising costs of 'high-tech' medicine, doctors can no longer separate clinical judgement from financial responsibility (Editorial, 1986). The cost of treatment must now be taken into account regardless of whether it is borne by the patient, the State or an insurance scheme. Admission to hospital is a major factor in keeping costs high and in Australia it is reported that the principal method of limiting costs in palliative cancer treatment is by reducing in-patient stay and the number of investigations, and by encouraging out-patient administration of chemotherapy (Friedlander and Tattersall, 1982).

Increased use of hospice services, particularly those providing home care, can also reduce total costs and, at the same time, increase the quality of compassionate care given to the patient. Again, visits by a home care nurse might be more useful than a long trip in an ambulance to see the doctor for psychological reasons (Rees, 1985).

The need to provide universally available treatment in the UK has led to rationing of resources, including less aggressive investigation of trivial complaints, less use of computerized tomography (CT) scanning, less intensive care beds in hospitals and less kidney dialysis in terminally ill patients (Aaron and Schwartz, 1985). British physicians are more comfortable than their American colleagues in rationing scarce resources such as hospital beds, and saying 'no' to some patients. It results in those resources becoming available to patients whose need is greater or in whom the resources are more likely to be effective. Physicians have always practised such discrimination even if the selection was usually subconscious.

The physician's attitude to the cost/benefit equation is often modified by the patient's expectations. An example is the observation that the expenditure per head on cytotoxic drugs in the UK is less than a quarter of that in the USA. It reflects different attitudes to the management of incurable cancer in the two countries. As expressed recently in an American journal: 'It is an American virtue to expect the best for oneself, and the present US health system responds to the national expectation by emphasizing high technology' (Cowan, 1986).

In Britain, until very recently, personal expectations have been more modest, and queuing for medical attention is part of the British system. If physicians in the UK accept the social obligation to provide equal access to health care for all, we must protect the system from breakdown by questioning the need for using the latest and most expensive technology in every case. Doctors concerned about the welfare of their patients are bound to be frustrated by the restraints imposed by rationing of resources, but this is the only way to give the best possible care to those who are most in need of it.

To summarize this section: it seems likely that technological innovation in medicine will increase progressively in coming years and that demand for its use will be insatiable. If good quality of care is to be freely available to all, restraint in costs is inevitable. In a private insurance-based system, cost containment is difficult but in a centrally controlled health service the best value for money must be pursued in order to release funds for new developments. This means some loss of autonomy for the clinician and more critical evaluation by his peers of clinical trials of new methods of diagnosis and treatment. Unfortunately, while most physicians in the UK are willing to practise self-restraint, some regard peer review and audit as a threat to their clinical freedom, rather than as an attempt to get better value for money.

WHAT PRICE QUALITY OF LIFE?

By definition, good palliative treatment should carry a high likelihood of rapidly relieving or preventing symptoms for a prolonged period. In addition it should take the minimum possible time to deliver the treatment and avoid iatrogenic symptoms. On the basis of this definition, a great deal of cancer treatment and investigation is over-aggressive and the best interests of the cancer patient are not always served. Yet, particularly in the USA, these procedures are often continued almost until the terminal stage, mainly 'to show the patient that a positive attempt is being made to retard the progress of the disease' (Stehlin and Beach, 1966).

These physicians claim that the use of cytotoxic therapy in advanced cancer has a second aim in addition to that of palliation—it *may* prolong life. The latter has been proved only in the case of leukaemia, lymphoma, trophoblastic tumours and some childhood tumours. For the majority of patients with moderately responsive cancer (response to chemotherapy in 40–75% of advanced cases), chemotherapy is palliative. There is often a significant survival advantage for responders over non-responders, but it is not possible to prove that this is a direct consequence of tumour response (Harding and Kaye, 1987). For those with poorly responsive tumours (response to chemotherapy in less than 40% of advanced cases) there is no conclusive evidence that survival benefit is related to tumour response.

Because we are unable to measure accurately the overall tumour response to treatment in late cancer, physicians are not clear as to which objectives are worth pursuing and which are not (Slevin, 1986). As an example, UICC criteria of response to systemic therapy in soft tissue lesions of breast cancer specify a minimum 50% decrease in the area of a lesion, which is equivalent to a mean decrease in diameter of about 30%. There are few patients to whom a reduction in a lump's diameter by one-third has anything but psychological value, particularly if its duration is a matter of a few months only. Even a possible prolongation of life by a month or two could hardly justify vitiating the quality of the patient's last few months of life. It is clear, therefore, that in the majority of cases the price is being paid by the patient for the privilege of maintaining hope.

There is no doubt that many patients need treatment for supportive reasons and an example of this is a reported series of patients with gastro-intestinal cancer who were treated by a 'low toxicity' combination of cytotoxic agents (Gough et al, 1981). Objective evidence of tumour regression was noted in only one out of the 25 cases treated, yet 23 of the patients and their relatives expressed their satisfaction with the treatment after completing three months of chemotherapy. The authors of the report conclude that the extra attention and psychological support reinforced 'the patients' subjective response to a chemotherapy protocol'. Surely a more valid conclusion was that the placebo chemotherapy helped to reinforce the patients' subjective response to the extra attention and psychological support. But was it necessary to use an expensive chemotherapy programme as a morale boosting placebo?

In selecting a palliative treatment the clinician must assess not only the likelihood of a response, but also its possible duration, promptness and degree of remission (Parbhoo, 1987). These factors must then be judged in the context of the estimated life expectation of the patient. Against these conjectural benefits must be set the more predictable factors, such as the side-effects of treatment, their effect on the patient's activity and their possible effects on the patient's mood. Travelling to and from hospital, repeated investigations and venepuncture must also be taken into account.

Every form of cancer treatment has a price in terms of morbidity. When palliation of local symptoms by radiotherapy is considered on this basis the balance sheet is relatively simple. One can usually promise that pain will be eased and a tumour reduced, and that, in the case of brain or mediastinal metastases, survival will almost certainly be prolonged as a result of relieving pressure by the tumour. The price to be paid is occasional radiation sickness, which is usually transient, predictable and easily countered.

But sometimes the equation is not so simple. Thus, if an advanced pelvic tumour is invading bladder or bowel, destruction of the tumour by radiation therapy is likely to lead to fistulae between organs, causing symptoms which are even more distressing than those of the original tumour. Again, if advanced pelvic tumour has obstructed the ureters and is causing uraemia, radiotherapy may relieve the obstruction and thereby gain a few extra months of life, but the patient may well suffer much more distressing symptoms before being overtaken by death (Bates, 1984).

The most widely used scale for assessing subjective benefit following treatment in advanced cancer is the *performance status* (Table 1), but the

Table 1. Classification of performance status.

Performance status (%)	Criteria
100	Normal, no complaints No evidence of disease
90	Able to carry on normal activity Minor signs or symptoms
80	Normal activity with effort Some signs or symptoms
70	Cares for self. Unable to carry on normal activity or to do active work
60	Requires occasional assistance, but able to care for most of needs
50	Requires considerable assistance and frequent medical care
40	Disabled and requires special care and assistance
30	Severely disabled. Hospitalization indicated but death not imminent
20	Very sick. Hospitalization and active supportive treatment necessary
10	Moribund

From Karnofsky and Burchenal (1948).

problem is that *quality of life* is almost impossible to measure. Self-rating questionnaires have been tried, although their disadvantage is that they are liable to be influenced by the image which the patient may wish to project, or thinks is expected. For this purpose, linear analogue self-assessment has been suggested (Priestman and Baum, 1976). In this method the patient marks along a series of scales the point most appropriate to each symptom or activity and the scores are added together to give an index. Serial assessments are possible and can be compared.

A major criticism is that all factors are given equal weighting in such an assessment. For example, a woman may suffer complete alopecia following treatment, but a fall in score on this account might be compensated for in the final total by an improved ability to do housework. How important is the latter compared to the former in assessing a patient's quality of life?

The problem of comparing different types of morbidity resulting from treatment is exemplified also in a recent report comparing mastectomy with breast conservation treatment (Fallowfield et al, 1986). While the mutilation resulting from mastectomy is assumed to be largely responsible for the high level of anxiety/depression common among treated breast cancer patients, the report found a similar level of stress in patients whose breast had been retained. It resulted from persisting anxiety about possible re-appearance of tumour in the treated breast. If informed consent is to be full, should we offer breast cancer patients a choice between the two types of anxiety?

It must be admitted that only too often the physician chooses the treatment based on his own particular training, his familiarity with a technique and his own personal attitudes to the side-effects. In the process he may minimize the disadvantages of the method he is advocating, perhaps unintentionally. One report notes that trained interviewers recognized toxicity following cytotoxic therapy in 90% of a group of patients while clinicians recognized it in only 60% of cases (Maguire et al, 1980).

In summary, therefore, all treatment for metastatic solid cancer is palliative and when several types of equally effective treatment are available, the less unpleasant methods should be offered first. Because such decisions are based on many imponderables, it may be useful to give some prime examples of inappropriate palliation:

- Aggressive treatment of asymptomatic metastases.
- The use of two methods in combination where one would be adequate.
- Prolonged duration of a palliative treatment in relation to the patient's life expectation.
- Severe morbidity from a treatment in relation to the degree of palliation which can be hoped for.

Motivation is obviously the major factor determining the acceptability of morbidity from treatment. If the patient assumes that the treatment is likely to help him individually he is more likely to regard morbidity as 'acceptable' than would a patient told he is taking part in a clinical trial. Such decisions are of course a function of age and personal attitudes to taking risks (Brewin, 1986). Whenever possible, the patient's attitude must prevail and in this connection it is important that the physician avoids pressure by relatives—one may hear very different wishes expressed by patients than those from their relatives.

COMMUNICATING WITH THE PATIENT

The physician who has to inform a patient that cancer has spread needs to realize that to some patients he appears to be delivering a death sentence. To all patients at this stage therefore the physician must offer hope. This often involves support of the patient's denial defence mechanisms. Patients should be given to understand that cancers behave differently in different people and that many patients with advanced cancer undergo remissions which may last for many years. Physical methods of treatment are also used, but they should not be given as a substitute for psychological support.

If the doctor's experience of the patient's particular manifestation makes him pessimistic, he may prefer to say little to the patient but this can lead to lack of empathy so that subsequent discussions involve only routine technical questions. Again, because detailed explanation is so time-consuming, physicians often talk in approximate half-truths, yet the patient may see from unconscious cues, such as a worried expression or awkward gaps of silence, that the physician is avoiding open discussion.

What do most cancer patients in the UK wish to know about the progress of their disease? There is obviously gross variation among patients according to social and cultural settings, and also according to individual attitudes of denial. It is even suggested that people vary from time to time in what they want to admit to themselves about their disease (Gyllenskold, 1982; Simpson, 1982). On this basis one cannot divide information-seekers from information-avoiders, but information must be given according to the patient's needs at that particular time. As a general rule one should give the patient only as much information as he asks for, can comprehend and can accept. In a study of hospital patients in the UK it was found that of those who suspected that they had cancer only one-third wanted to know the prognosis. No patient wanted to know if the disease was likely to prove fatal (McIntosh, 1976).

The patient should, however, be given an informed choice of treatment wherever possible and we noted above that his decision may well differ from that of the family. It will obviously depend on his general condition and attitude to the side-effects and morbidity of active treatment, whether by surgery, radiotherapy or cytotoxic therapy. If choices are difficult, the patient with advanced disease should not be confronted for a decision, because patients' wishes can often be deduced by careful listening by the carers.

Most patients, especially younger patients, prefer the doctor to act as an adviser rather than take an authoritative role. It may be that the patient's feeling of helplessness in the face of cancer is counteracted by improving his knowledge and involving him in the decision-taking process; but there is considerable difficulty in explaining even to a highly intelligent patient the gross uncertainties of both cancer growth and its treatment. The widespread practice of informed consent in the USA is probably due less to alteration in social opinion on the rights of patients than to changes in legal requirements and malpractice suits.

It is relevant to compare two reports from the USA. The first (Cassileth et al, 1980) suggested that 87% of younger cancer patients wanted full participation in the doctor's decision, compared with 51% of older patients. Only about 10% of all patients wanted no information at all and another 10% wanted only minimal or optimistic information. Yet, in another series in the USA (Leigh et al, 1980), it was found that in a group of 100 patients who were all told of their diagnosis of cancer before being treated, subsequent questioning showed that 48% of men and 16% of women denied that they were aware of the diagnosis. In addition, 81% of the men and 63% of the women regarded their illness as not being severe in spite of the information they had received!

Most doctors would agree that it is counterproductive and unnecessary to inform the patient of every possible complication of treatment, as has become the norm in the USA for medicolegal reasons. Similarly, it is confusing to discuss conjectural benefits of one treatment against another and the various controversies in medical opinion. Rather than discuss possible duration of survival, it is better to couch the prognosis in terms of percentage chance of either cure or palliation of symptoms. Promises such as 'there is a 90% chance that chemotherapy will be successful' are commonly given to patients with only moderately sensitive solid cancers such as breast cancer. While these promises may give the patient hope, they make it difficult for her to refuse unpleasant treatment because the patient wrongly assumes that 'success' means prolongation of survival.

The appearance of each new manifestation of cancer creates a sense of despair in the patient and is also a psychological blow to the physician aiming to maintain hope in the patient. Every patient will require reassurance and encouraging explanation with each new complication. It is important at this stage that the patient sets himself day-by-day goals which can actually be realized (Calman, 1984), and that the physician keeps the patient ambulatory and out of hospital for as long as possible.

Not all patients cope mentally by adjusting to, and accepting, the threat to life. Denial attitudes are more common than was previously thought and are said to persist in up to 20% of cases (Simpson, 1982). Denial is not an all-or-none phenomenon nor should it be regarded as abnormal. It is part of the psychological defences of each individual and, under normal circumstances, should be supported by the physician. As noted above, seemingly intelligent people may insist on denying that they are suffering from cancer even after having been told the diagnosis, and such denial should not be discouraged (Hughes, 1986).

The most likely time for emotional breakdown, apart from the time of diagnosis, is at the first appearance of recurrence or metastasis. It is claimed that the patient at high risk to breakdown may be recognized by certain psychosocial characteristics: history of failure to cope in the presence of stress; evidence of psychological instability or a history of a multiproblem background; low socio-economic status or little moral support from those around (Lee, 1986).

It has been commented that complaints of anxiety or depression are recorded by physicians in only a very small proportion of case histories of cancer patients (Silberfarb, 1986). One factor is that most patients believe that symptoms of anxiety will be regarded as a sign of inadequacy or weakness. As a result their complaints tend to refer to more socially acceptable reasons for loss of self-confidence, such as mutilation from surgery, amputation, mastectomy, laryngectomy or colostomy.

A possible second reason why cancer patients rarely mention their psychological problems to their doctors is that they regard them as too busy and involved only with their physical well-being. Disclosure of toxic symptoms to a surgeon was found to be considerably less than to an oncologist, the conclusion being that patients avoid complaining to some of their medical attendants, either for fear of losing their sympathy or because communication barriers are greater (Buckman, 1986).

A third reason is that doctors do not enquire too specifically about the patient's peace of mind. It is said that less than 1% of communication between doctor and patient is concerned with the patient's emotional reaction to the diagnosis of cancer or its complications (Maguire et al, 1974). Yet, it has been stressed that cancer patients need to work through their anxiety, just as bereaved people need to work through their mourning.

The problem is that physicians have to fulfil a double role in their management of the patient with advanced cancer (Gyllenskold, 1982). First, they need an objective and detached attitude if they are to put the patient through a series of unpleasant tests or treatments. Second, they need an understanding of the patient's anxieties without loss of self-identity. Many physicians unfortunately find it difficult to alternate between the two roles. If they cannot put themselves in the patient's place they are unhappy and out of their depth when called upon for psychological support of the cancer patient. The clinician's task involves not only problem-solving, decision-making and technical knowledge, but also sensitivity to the emotional state of the patient and providing moral support, and doctors are clearly not equal in their capacity to demonstrate compassion, understanding and support in a tangible form. Sometimes, too, the 'chemistry' between doctor and patient may not be right; doctors and patients rarely choose each other.

The medical student sees little of the team care necessary in the management of the cancer patient—particularly of the late cancer patient. Doctors are rarely trained in the psychological management of severe illness and often feel helpless when faced with the psychological, family and social problems of the cancer patient. They may try to ignore them or else compensate for a feeling of inadequacy by showing professional over-activity. Such busy behaviour often satisfies the family members who wish to be reassured that no stone has been left unturned. It usually fails to meet the needs of the patient.

Most clinicians, and indeed many medical personnel, including nurses, become paternalistic in their behaviour to the patient and tend to make decisions on behalf of patients. Indeed, many would argue that it is cruel to ask the patient to take difficult medical decisions and that the patient is not qualified to judge the situation objectively (Gillon, 1981). They believe that the majority of patients expect their physicians to take full responsibility and that paternalism and domination are essential for the physician's effectiveness. They may list alternative treatments to the patient but will still recommend a specific choice. They think it unethical to say 'go ahead and choose, it's your life' (Ingelfinger, 1980).

However, there are dangers. The technical training of physicians lays increasing stress on machine-controlled survival and spare part surgery. But should we fight incessantly to add months to the cancer patient's life or should we fight for good quality life only? It depends on whether the patient is a risk-taker by nature, and only the patient can make the decision. The physician, for his part, requires a wide experience of the disease and considerable clinical judgement. These, combined with a sense of compassion, will enable him to steer the patient to a decision best suited to the individual and his disease.

THE TERMINAL STAGE

The patient with advanced cancer not only has to contend with physical symptoms but also has to cope emotionally with the threat of dying. The degree of this additional anxiety is often related to the tempo at which the disease is progressing (Hoy, 1987). As patients' dependence on treatment increases, so their anxiety tends to focus on possible ways in which they may die (e.g. choking, suffocating, pain, paralysis, etc.). It is at this stage especially that the physician has to extend himself to provide hopefulness and compassionate care. Even if he cannot prolong survival he can offer physical comfort, and his reassurance can play as crucial a role as the physical treatment which he provides.

When terminal care is the goal, investigations must be restricted to those which will improve symptom control. When attempts to prolong life are still appropriate, active treatment is justified only after discussing the probable morbidity and possible duration of response with the family and patient. Unproven treatments should be used only as part of a carefully controlled clinical trial, and even then, only at the request of the patient and relatives. Cytotoxic therapy should in general be withheld from elderly patients with widely disseminated disease and in poor condition.

The duration of a palliative treatment must be commensurate with the patient's life expectation. It is not justifiable to occupy the last few weeks or months of a patient's life with a prolonged course of active therapy in a hospital. Death of a cancer patient in the middle of a course of treatment (whether radiotherapy or cytotoxic agents) can be justified if the treatment is an attempt at cure and a calculated risk is being taken. If, however, a patient dies in the middle of palliative treatment, it may indicate poor clinical judgement on the part of the physician.

In extenuation it is sometimes suggested that a decision to treat has been forced by the patient or relatives demanding that no stone be left unturned. But the hopes of the latter are often unrealistic and it is clear that our duty is to the patient and not to assuage relatives. We should not feel guilty if we do not offer technically complex treatments in this highly scientific age but it often takes more time to explain why we do not advise it than it takes to arrange such treatment.

There comes a time when aggressive treatment is no longer appropriate. The physician's need to treat and the family's need to treat are unacceptable reasons for active therapy (Mount, 1978). It is important to explain to the family that the stage is *not* one where 'nothing more can be done', even if therapy can no longer control the disease progress. The only goal is now to alleviate suffering because nothing can be done to prolong life without too great a cost in side-effects. In the USA there is a tendency to be more aggressive in the management of the terminally ill patient. Procedures such as prolonged artificial nutrition, aggressive cytotoxic therapy and cardio-pulmonary resuscitation are not uncommonly used for such patients. Such procedures would be rarely employed in the UK.

There is a need to mention physicians' personal attitude to death. Few people have enough insight to evaluate their own prejudices and, in the case of the physician, this may present problems in the management of the pre-terminal cancer patient. One of the symptoms of our modern detribalized society is that we are unable to cope confidently with death. Mere discussion of the process of dying and interment makes most of us feel awkward and inadequate. It has been said that physicians can help patients face their fears only if they are able to recognize their own.

In the last 80 years death has become institutionalized, and about 60% of all people now die in hospital, often with tubes attached to every orifice. Death is hardly mentioned in our medical institutions, yet a recent report (Hinton, 1980) suggests that a majority of pre-terminal cancer patients are aware of their condition. Over one-third experience distressing symptoms of anxiety or depression, and the figure is even higher in patients under 50 who feel also angry and cheated. About three-quarters of late cancer patients are said to recognize that they might die soon and speak of this to their spouses or to medical personnel, and it appears to be rare for patients to maintain denial to the end (Kubler Ross, 1969).

Should cancer patients be told they are dying? Such information should clearly be withheld if it might cause despair, but evasion of the truth is usually detected. Blank denial of an obvious prognosis will increase the patient's fears and destroy his trust in the physician. But, equally, there is no place for confronting the patient with undesired information. Optimism and hope must be encouraged and most would agree that a question such as 'when am I going to die?' should not be accepted literally because it is an expression of the patient's fears, rather than a desire for knowledge (Luce, 1979). It has been stressed that terminal patients are less likely to experience anxiety or depression if they can discuss their problems (Hinton, 1980). But the patient's willingness to talk about death depends on whether others are prepared to listen and talk about this awareness.

CONCLUSION

There is no firm evidence that aggressive systemic therapy and its associated wearying investigations prolong life in the vast majority of patients with advanced solid cancer. Yet they are capable of vitiating the patient's quality of survival. Palliative therapy should therefore proceed sequentially, the less unpleasant methods being offered first. Some prime examples of inappropriate palliation are: aggressive cytotoxic treatment of asymptomatic metastases in moderately or poorly sensitive tumours; the use of two methods of treatment in combination where one would be adequate; prolonged duration of a palliative treatment in relation to the patient's life expectation; severe morbidity from a treatment in relation to the degree of palliation which can be hoped for.

Because of advances in cancer treatment, patients now live longer and suffer for a longer time than they did in the past. The previous chapters have clearly shown that our ability to control distressing symptoms has also progressed enormously, whether in the early, advanced or palliative phases of cancer. Unfortunately, however, such care is not widely practised by physicians who are preoccupied by active curative or palliative treatment. It tends to be delegated to a junior assistant because it is often regarded as secondary to the more important aim of tumour control.

It is essential that control of distressing symptoms always runs prominently alongside other forms of cancer treatment. In the case of aggressive treatment aiming at cure, the treatment itself may cause the distressing symptoms. Their relief cannot be regarded as incidental to the main goal, but must be an integral part of the development of new aggressive techniques. In the case of palliative treatment, there is a tendency to offer the patient promise of relief of distressing symptoms when tumour regression has been achieved. Such delay is unjustifiable in most cases, and each goal must be pursued separately although the paths may run parallel. Finally, in the case of terminal management, relief of distressing symptoms is the only rational aim for a physician who is part of a team devoted to the whole of the patient's welfare. It is part of the physician's unwritten contract with the cancer patient.

REFERENCES

Aaron HJ & Schwartz WB (1985) *The Painful Prescription; Rationing Hospital Care*. Washington: The Brookings Institution.

Bates T (1984) Radiotherapy in terminal care. In Saunders C (ed.) *The Management of Terminal Malignant Disease*. London: Edward Arnold.

Brewin TB (1986) Quality of survival. In Stoll BA (ed.) *Coping with Cancer Stress*, p 83. Dordrecht: Martinus Nijhoff.

Buckman R (1986) Communicating with the patient. In Stoll BA (ed.) *Coping with Cancer Stress*, p 167. Dordrecht: Martinus Nijhoff.

Calman KC (1984) Quality of life in cancer patients—an hypothesis. *Journal of Medical Ethics* **10:** 124–127.

Cassileth BR, Zupkis RV, Sutton Smith K et al (1980) Information on participation preferences among cancer patients. *Annals of Internal Medicine* **92:** 832–839.

Cowan JA (1986) Administrative waste in US health care. *New England Journal of Medicine* **315:** 1034.

Editorial (1986) Improving use of clinical resources. *Lancet* **ii:** 319–320.

Editorial (1987) The controlled clinical trial; consensus? *Lancet* **ii:** 547.

Fallowfield LJ, Baum M & Maguire GP (1986) Breast conservation and psychological morbidity associated with diagnosis and treatment of early breast cancer. *British Medical Journal* **293:** 1331–1334.

Friedlander ML & Tattersall MHN (1982) Counting the costs of cancer therapy. *European Journal of Cancer and Clinical Oncology* **18:** 1237–1241.

Gillon R (1981) The function of criticism. *British Medical Journal* **283:** 1633–1634.

Gough IR, Furnival CM & Butnett W (1981) Patient attitudes to chemotherapy for advanced gastrointestinal cancer. *Clinical Oncology* **7:** 5–10.

Gyllenskold K (1982) *Breast Cancer. The Psychological Effect of the Disease and its Treatment*, p 84. London: Tavistock Publications.

Harding M & Kaye SB (1987) Prognostic significance of response to therapy. In Stoll BA (ed.) *Pointers to Cancer Prognosis*, p 65. Dordrecht: Martinus Nijhoff.

Hinton J (1980) Whom do dying patients tell? *British Medical Journal* **281:** 1328–1331.

Hoy AM (1987) Clinical pointers to prognosis in terminal disease. In Stoll BA (ed.) *Pointers to Cancer Prognosis*, p 79. Dordrecht: Martinus Nijhoff.

Hughes J (1986) Denial in cancer patients. In Stoll BA (ed.) *Coping with Cancer Stress*, p 63. Dordrecht: Martinus Nijhoff.

Ingelfinger F (1980) Arrogance. *New England Journal of Medicine* **303:** 1507–1509.

Karnofsky DA & Burchenal JH (1948) In MacLeod CM (ed.) *Evaluation of Chemotherapeutic Agents*, p 101. New York: Columbia University Press.

Klein R (1984) Rationing health care. *British Medical Journal* **289:** 143–144.

Kubler Ross E (1969) *On Death and Dying*. New York: Macmillan.

Lee MS (1986) Monitoring of coping. In Stoll BA (ed.) *Coping with Cancer Stress*, p 113. Dordrecht: Martinus Nijhoff.

Leigh H, Ungerer J & Percarpio B (1980) Denial and helplessness in cancer patients undergoing radiation therapy. *Cancer* **45:** 3086–3089.
Luce JK (1979) Selecting patients for supportive therapy. In Stoll BA (ed.) *Mind and Cancer Prognosis*, p 127. Chichester: John Wiley.
McIntosh J (1976) Patients' awareness and desire for information about diagnosed but undisclosed malignant disease. *Lancet* **ii:** 300–302.
Maguire GP, Julier DL, Kawton KE & Bancroft JHJ (1974) Psychiatric morbidity and referral on two general medical wards. *British Medical Journal* **1:** 268–271.
Maguire GP, Tait A, Brooke M et al (1980) Psychiatric morbidity and physical toxicity associated with adjuvant chemotherapy after mastectomy. *British Medical Journal* **281:** 1179–1183.
Mount BM (1978) Palliative care of the patient with terminal cancer. In Skinner DG & de Kenion JB (eds) *Genitourinary Cancer*, p 535. Philadelphia: WB Saunders.
Parbhoo SP (1987) Clinical pointers to rapid growth. In Stoll BA (ed.) *Pointers to Cancer Prognosis*, p 3. Dordrecht: Martinus Nijhoff.
Priestman TJ & Baum M (1976) Evaluation of quality of life for patients receiving treatment for advanced breast cancer. *Lancet* **i:** 899–901.
Rees GJ (1985) Cost effectiveness in oncology. *Lancet* **ii:** 1405–1408.
Silberfarb PM (1986) Psychological impact on the patient. In Stoll BA (ed.) *Breast Cancer; Treatment and Prognosis*, p 98. Oxford: Blackwell Scientific Publications.
Silbermann HR (1986) Minimising economic hardships of diagnosis and treatment. In Laszlo J (ed.) *Physician's Guide to Cancer Care Complications*, p 15. New York: Marcel Dekker.
Simpson MA (1982) Therapeutic uses of truth. In Wilkes E (ed.) *The Dying Patient*, p 255. Lancaster: MTP Press.
Slevin ML (1986) Assessing response to systemic therapy. In Stoll BA (ed.) *Breast Cancer; Treatment and Prognosis*, p 264. Oxford: Blackwell Scientific.
Stehlin JS & Beach KH (1966) Psychological aspects of cancer therapy. *Journal of the American Medical Association* **197:** 140–148.

Index

Note: Page numbers of article titles are in **bold** type.